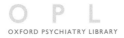

O P L
OXFORD PSYCHIATRY LIBRARY

Generalized Anxiety Disorder

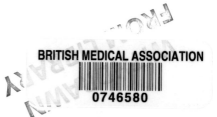

► Except where otherwise stated, drug doses and recommendations are for the non-pregnant adult who is not breastfeeding.

► Some of the medication and dosages suggested in this book are outside of the usual licensed indications and dosage ranges, however they are suggested as a result of utilizing trial evidence and the specialists with expertise in the subject area. Some of the medication discussed in the book is not available in the UK, but may be widely used in another country and has been included for completeness

O P L
OXFORD PSYCHIATRY LIBRARY

Generalized Anxiety Disorder

Michael Van Ameringen

Professor, Department of Psychiatry and
Behavioural Neurosciences
McMaster University,
Hamilton, Ontario, Canada

Mark H. Pollack

Grainger Professor and Chairman
Department of Psychiatry
Rush University Medical Center
Chicago, USA

OXFORD
UNIVERSITY PRESS

OXFORD
UNIVERSITY PRESS

Great Clarendon Street, Oxford OX2 6DP

Oxford University Press is a department of the University of Oxford.
It furthers the University's objective of excellence in research, scholarship,
and education by publishing worldwide in

Oxford New York

Auckland Cape Town Dar es Salaam Hong Kong Karachi
Kuala Lumpur Madrid Melbourne Mexico City Nairobi
New Delhi Shanghai Taipei Toronto

With offices in

Argentina Austria Brazil Chile Czech Republic France Greece
Guatemala Hungary Italy Japan Poland Portugal Singapore
South Korea Switzerland Thailand Turkey Ukraine Vietnam

Oxford is a registered trade mark of Oxford University Press
in the UK and in certain other countries

Published in the United States
by Oxford University Press Inc., New York

British Library Cataloguing in Publication Data

Data available

Library of Congress Cataloging in Publication Data

Data available

Typeset by Newgen Imaging Systems (P) Ltd., Chennai, India
Printed in Great Britain
on acid-free paper by
Ashford Colour Press Ltd, Gosport, Hampshire

ISBN 978-0-19-955783-7

10 9 8 7 6 5 4 3 2

Whilst every effort has been made to ensure that the contents of this book are as
complete, accurate and up-to-date as possible at the date of writing. Oxford
University Press is not able to give any guarantee or assurance that such is the case.
Readers are urged to take appropriately qualified medical advice in all cases. The
information in this book is intended to be useful to the general reader, but should
not be used as a means of self-diagnosis or for the prescription of medication.

Contents

Contributors

Catherine Mancini
Associate Professor
Department of Psychiatry and
Behavioural Neurosciences
McMaster University;
Hamilton, Ontario, Canada

Beth Patterson
Department of Psychiatry and
Behavioural Neurosciences,
McMaster University;
Hamilton, Ontario, Canada

Mark H. Pollack
Grainger Professor
and Chairman
Department of Psychiatry
Rush University Medical Center
Chicago, USA

Michael Van Ameringen
Professor,
Department of Psychiatry and
Behavioural Neurosciences
McMaster University,
Hamilton, Ontario
Canada

Abbreviations

ACC	anterior cingulate cortex
ACTH	adrenocorticotropic hormone (corticotropin)
ADHD	attention deficit hyperactivity disorder
CBT	cognitive behavioural therapy
CNS	central nervous system
CRH	corticotropin-releasing hormone
DBPC	double-blind placebo-controlled study
DBS	deep brain stimulation
DSM	Diagnostic and Statistical Manual
ECG	electrocardiogram
ECT	electroconvulsive therapy
EPS	extra-pyramidal symptoms
ERP	exposure and response prevention
fMRI	functional magnetic resonance imaging
GABA	gamma-aminobutyric acid
GAD	generalized anxiety disorder
HAMA	Hamilton Anxiety Rating Scale
5-HT	5-hydroxytryptamine
ICD	International Classification of Diseases
MAOI	monoamine oxidase inhibitor
MASC	Multidimensional Anxiety Scale for Children
MDD	major depressive disorder
MIDUS	Midlife Development in the United States
mPFC	medial prefrontal cortex
mPFG	medial prefrontal gyrus
m/r	modified release
NARI	noradrenaline (norepinephrine) reuptake inhibitor
NaSSA	noradrenergic and specific serotonergic antidepressant
NCS-R	National Comorbidity Survey Replication
OCD	obsessive-compulsive disorder
PCC	posterior cingulate cortex
PD	panic disorder
PTSD	post-traumatic stress disorder

RCT	randomized controlled trial
RIMA	reversible inhibitor of monoamine oxidase A
rTMS	repetitive transcranial magnetic stimulation
SAD	social anxiety disorder (social phobia)
SCARED	Screen for Child Anxiety Related Disorders
SGRI	selective GABA reuptake inhibitor
SNRI	serotonin noradrenaline re-uptake inhibitor
SSRI	selective serotonin re-uptake inhibitor
TCA	tricyclic antidepressant
TD	tardive dyskinesia

Chapter 1

Introduction

Michael Van Ameringen and Mark H. Pollack

The clinical entity of generalized anxiety disorder (GAD) has evolved considerably since its inclusion in the third edition of the *Diagnostic and Statistical Manual* (DSM III) in 1980. It initially emerged as a residual diagnostic category and has become a distinct psychiatric disorder in DSM IV and *International Classification of Diseases* (tenth revision-ICD-10). GAD is one of the most common anxiety disorders, afflicting about 6% of the general population in their lifetime and is even more prevalent in primary care settings. It is associated with high rates of psychiatric co-morbidity particularly major depressive disorder and other anxiety disorders as well as with medical co-morbidity. GAD patients often present with chronic, somatic complaints and are high utilizers of medical services. The prominence of the somatic symptoms manifested by many of these patients may obscure the underlying anxiety disorder and present a diagnostic challenge for clinicians. GAD was initially felt to be a mild condition causing minimal impairment in functioning; however, more recent evidence suggests that the burden associated with GAD is broad and encompasses impairment in psychological, social, and occupational functioning and an overall decreased quality of life.

Our understanding of the aetiology of this disorder is at its infancy; however, preliminary findings in the area of neurobiology, neuro-imaging, and molecular genetics have implicated the involvement of critical CNS systems including key brain structures such as the insula and amygdala.

Extensive systematic study supports the efficacy of pharmacotherapy and psychosocial interventions for the treatment of GAD. Extensive work has been done examining a wide variety of medications in the treatment of GAD. Antidepressants, anxiolytics, anticonvulsants, antipsychotics, and antihistamines have all been shown to be efficacious as GAD treatments. Psychotherapy, in the form of a number of variations of cognitive and cognitive-behavioural therapy (CBT), has also been shown to be effective for GAD.

The course of GAD can be both chronic and episodic, requiring a long-term treatment approach. Unfortunately, there is little information to guide clinicians in this area. Although many patients respond at least somewhat to an initial treatment intervention, achieving and maintaining remission can be more difficult. It is unclear whether treating GAD prevents common sequelae such as the development of co-morbid depression, although some indirect evidence suggests it might. There is also little guidance available as to next-step treatments after initial treatments fail. Although GAD is the only anxiety disorder that increases in prevalence with advancing age, more work needs to be done to evaluate the treatment of GAD in the elderly.

Despite the existence of evidence-based treatments, many affected individuals do not have ready access to them, particularly empirically based CBT. Moreover, even evidence-based treatments are often not delivered in accordance to recommended treatment guidelines, resulting in sub-optimal outcomes. As a field, we need to improve our dissemination of these evidence-based treatments so that they are administered in a variety of health-care settings.

In this book, we have summarized research findings in GAD in order to provide the reader with a broad understanding of the disorder. This background information has been integrated with a practical 'how-to' approach for treating patients who suffer from this highly prevalent and impairing disorder. Helpful treatment resources for both clinicians and patients have been provided and it is our hope that the information in this book will lead to better treatment outcomes for individuals who suffer from GAD.

Chapter 2

Diagnosis and prevalence

Beth Patterson, Michael Van Ameringen,
and Mark H. Pollack

> ## Key points
>
> - The diagnostic criteria for generalized anxiety disorder (GAD) have evolved considerably since its inception.
> - *Diagnostic and Statistical Manual* (DSM)-IV-TR and *International Classification of Diseases* (ICD)-10 both diagnose similar rates of GAD, in spite of different criteria.
> - Worldwide rates of lifetime DSM-IV GAD range from 2.3% to 5.7%.

2.1 Diagnostic classification

The characterization of generalized anxiety disorder (GAD) has been the subject of substantial debate since its inception. Sigmund Freud described the symptoms of GAD ~100 yrs ago when he separated 'anxiety neurosis' from 'neurasthenia', a term coined by neurologists George Beard and S. Weir Mitchell to describe a culturally oriented diagnosis that attributed mental and physical symptoms to the lack of nervous energy brought on by the stresses of modern society. Freud used 'neurasthenia' more broadly to characterize general lassitude, irritability, lack of concentration, worry, and hypochondria. According to Freud, there were four main components of anxiety neurosis, including general irritability, anxiety attacks, secondary phobic avoidance, and 'anxious expectation', which involved nervousness, apprehension, and free-floating anxiety: hallmark symptoms of currently defined GAD (Rickels and Rynn 2001).

The *Diagnostic and Statistical Manual of Mental Disorders*, or DSM, is the primary classification system used for mental disorders in North America. The concept of 'neurosis' as the major defining principle in the classification of the anxiety disorders was used in both the first and second editions of the DSM (DSM-I and DSM-II), published in 1952 and 1968, respectively, and was based on the belief, as influenced by psychoanalytic theory and practice, that all psychopathology was secondary to anxiety.

The actual diagnosis of GAD appeared for the first time in DSM-III, published in 1980. DSM-III represented a significant shift from the psychoanalytic principles of anxiety neurosis, which characterized DSM-I and II to a more empirical approach where psychiatric disorders were defined in terms of age of onset, duration of illness, and symptom severity and patterns.

In DSM-III, anxiety neurosis actually was subdivided into two categories:

1. GAD, defined with a 1-month duration criterion, and included anxious patients with no, or few, panic attacks and no phobic avoidance

2. Panic disorder specified by number of panic attacks (phobic avoidance).

This schema was based to some extent on a so-called 'pharmacological dissection' of anxiety derived from studies of drug response in the 1960s and 1970s in panic and phobic disorders which suggested that imipramine was beneficial in patients who had spontaneous panic attacks and in those who had panic attacks with phobic avoidance but not in subjects with severe generalized anxiety and no phobic avoidance or in subjects with simple phobias and no panic attacks (Klein and Klein 1990) and that benzodiazepines were more effective for non-panic generalized anxiety. Although this conceptualization broke down in the 1980s when it was demonstrated that the benzodiazepine alprazolam was effective for panic disorder (American Psychiatric Association 1987) and that the tricyclic antidepressant imipramine was effective for GAD. The DSM-III criteria for GAD was criticized as lacking specifically defined symptomatology and led to inconsistent and unreliable diagnosis and inflated estimates of the prevalence rate of GAD. The DSM-III-R (American Psychiatric Association 1987) re-defined GAD so that the duration criterion was extended to 6 months, but still included the concept of 'anxiety neurosis'. DSM-III-R GAD was difficult to diagnose, however, due to its broadly somatic nature. Many other mood and anxiety disorders shared similar somatic symptoms with GAD and there seemed to be no one cardinal psychologic, behavioural, or somatic symptom to distinguish GAD from other disorders. In 1993, Marten and colleagues (1993) examined the symptom criterion for GAD and assisted in setting the framework for DSM-IV with their finding that seven of the original 18 symptoms could be identified as hallmark symptoms consistently present in GAD. The authors also recommended that the cardinal symptom of 'unrealistic worry' be refined to uncontrollable worry in order to better distinguish GAD from non-anxious individuals. In the DSM-IV (American Psychiatric Association 1994), GAD was further refined to reflect the research-based concept that anxiety is a product of the interaction of neurobiology, psychological and psychosocial factors, and environmental stressors. The 6-month duration criterion was maintained however, GAD was classified as a separate anxiety disorder alongside panic disorder, agoraphobia, social phobia, specific phobia, obsessive–compulsive disorder, acute stress disorder, and post-traumatic stress disorder. The term 'neurosis' was disbanded in this iteration of DSM. In the most recent edition of the DSM, DSM-IV-Text Revision (TR), the diagnostic criteria were unchanged from DSM-IV (Table 2.1).

The tenth revision of the *International Classification of Diseases* (ICD-10) (World Health Organization 1992) is used most frequently in Europe for diagnostic classification. It is largely consistent with the DSM-IV criteria for GAD, although the ICD-10 uses more 'flexible' phraseology, making the classification somewhat more loosely defined than DSM-IV. The prominent feature of the ICD-10 classification for GAD is that anxiety is generalized and persistent and not restricted

Table 2.1 DSM-IV-TR (American Psychiatric Association 2000)

1. Excessive anxiety and worry (apprehensive expectation) occurring more days than not for at least 6 months, about a number of events or activities (such as work or school performance)

2. The person finds it difficult to control the worry

3. The anxiety and worry are associated with three (or more) of the following six symptoms (with at least some symptoms present for more days than not for the past 6 months):

   a) Restlessness or feeling keyed up or on edge

   b) Being easily fatigued

   c) Difficulty concentrating or mind going blank

   d) Irritability

   e) Muscle tension

   f) Sleep disturbances (difficulty falling or staying asleep, or restless unsatisfying sleep)

4. The focus of the anxiety and worry is not confined to the features of an Axis 1 disorder and the anxiety and worry do not occur exclusively during post-traumatic stress disorder

5. The anxiety, worry, or physical symptoms cause clinically significant distress or impairment in social, occupational, or other important areas of functioning

6. The disturbance is not due to the direct physiological effects of a substance or a general medical condition and does not occur exclusively during a mood disorder, a psychotic disorder, or a pervasive developmental disorder

to any particular environmental circumstances. Primary symptoms of anxiety must be present most days for at least several weeks at a time, and usually for several months. These symptoms should usually involve elements of apprehension, motor tension, and autonomic activity. In ICD-10, GAD is considered to be a residual diagnosis such that a patient may not meet full diagnostic criteria for it if they also meet criteria for other anxiety disorders or depression (although the transient appearance of other symptoms is acceptable). Table 2.2 highlights the diagnostic criteria for GAD in ICD-10.

There are several key differences between DSM-IV and ICD-10 when diagnosing GAD. These are summarized in Table 2.3.

Table 2.2 ICD-10 (World Health Organization 1992)

1. There must have been a period of at least 6 months with prominent tension, worry, and feelings of apprehension about everyday events and problems
2. At least four of the following symptoms listed below must be present at least one of which must be from items 1 to 4

Autonomic arousal symptoms

1. Palpitations or pounding heat or accelerated heart rate
2. Sweating
3. Trembling or shaking
4. Dry mouth (not due to medication or dehydration)

Symptoms involving chest or abdomen

5. Difficulty in breathing
6. Feeling of choking
7. Chest pain or discomfort
8. Nausea or abdominal distress (e.g. churning stomach)

Symptoms involving mental state

9. Feeling dizzy, unsteady, faint, or light-headed
10. Feeling that objects are unreal (derealization) or that the self is distant or 'not really here' (depersonalization)
11. Fear of losing control, 'going crazy', or passing out
12. Fear of dying

General symptoms

13. Hot flashes or cold chills
14. Numbness or tingling sensations

Symptoms of tension

15. Muscle tension or aches and pains
16. Restlessness and inability to relax
17. Feeling keyed up, on edge, or mentally tense
18. Sensation of lump in the throat, or difficulty in swallowing

Other non-specific symptoms

19. Exaggerated response to minor surprises or being startled
20. Difficulty in concentrating or mind going blank
21. Persistent irritability
22. Difficulty in getting to sleep because of worrying

Table 2.3 Key differences between DSM-IV and ICD-10 diagnostic criteria for GAD

	DSM-IV	ICD-10
Diagnostic classification	Independent category	Residual category
Worry/anxiety symptom	Excessive anxiety and worry	Persistent free-floating anxiety
Duration	≥6 months	Several months
Autonomic hyperactivity and psychic symptoms	Not essential	Must be present
Functional impairment	Must be present	Not specified

Both ICD-10 and DSM-IV require that persistent anxiety or worry is present for a considerable time; however, in DSM-IV the anxiety and worry is 'excessive' and in ICD-10 it is persistent and free floating. Both systems include physical and/or psychic symptoms to be present; however, only ICD-10 mandates that symptoms of autonomic hyperactivity, such as tachycardia, sweating, light-headedness, are present.

Slade and Andrews (2001) used data of 10,641 respondents in the Australian National Survey of Health and Wellbeing to compare the diagnostic classification systems of DSM-IV and ICD-10. The rates of diagnosed GAD were similar with both schedules: the 12-month rate was 2.6% when using DSM-IV and 3.0% when using ICD-10. The authors examined specific diagnostic criteria and concluded that though the overall rates were similar, the instruments identified somewhat different patients. ICD-10 GAD identifies a more somatic, less disabling form of the condition than DSM-IV GAD which focuses more on cognitive symptomatology and has a higher weighting on 'excessiveness' and 'distress'. It is currently unclear what will become of GAD in the next iteration of the DSM, DSM-V. Although there is a push to achieve more cohesion between the DSM and ICD diagnostic systems, one of the primary issues regarding the reclassification of GAD lies in its similarities to major depressive disorder (MDD). As will be described in a subsequent section of this book, there is a high degree of co-morbidity between MDD and GAD. It has been argued that current diagnostic classification systems cannot account for such phenomena as the systems are too heavily based upon the assumption that disorders within a particular category (e.g. anxiety disorders) are more strongly related than those in separate categories. Disorders are currently grouped according to their diagnostic and clinical features (phenomenology), but this may not take into consideration what has been found in empirical, genetic, and clinical data. Empirical evidence derived from studies of epidemiology have shown high correlations between GAD and MDD and in structural modelling studies, there has been a high degree of association between the two disorders, especially with regard to the factor of negative affectivity.

In some studies there is significant genotypic overlap between GAD and MDD (Mennin *et al.* 2008). Clinically, both disorders respond well to treatment with selective serotonin reuptake inhibitors (SSRIs) and serotonin norepinephrine reuptake inhibitors (SNRIs), further suggesting a strong relationship.

It has been suggested that based on these compelling similarities, GAD and MDD should be grouped together in DSM-V, along with dysthymia, post-traumatic stress disorder, and neurasthenia as part of a group of disorders characterized by 'distress' (two other categories, 'fear' and 'externalizing' disorders are also proposed in this model [Andrews *et al.* 2008]). Other suggestions for changes to DSM-V have included: re-categorizing GAD as a mood disorder, subsuming GAD under MDD as a subtype much like agitated depression, or using a broader category such as neuroticism to describe both disorders (Mennin *et al.* 2008).

Other researchers have argued that although there are similarities between GAD and MDD, there are equally compelling differences, making the removal of GAD as a separate diagnosis and subsuming it under MDD premature. In a paper by Mennin and colleagues (2008), the authors argue that GAD shares a much more complex relationship with mood and anxiety disorders and that any re-classification of this disorder needs to take into account factors such as the established reliability and validity of GAD as a separate diagnosis, that MDD also overlaps substantially with other anxiety disorders and that although GAD and MDD share similar genetics, they can be differentiated by environmental factors and temporal presentations.

Field trials are currently underway as the architects of DSM-V examine proposed revisions for the classification of GAD (Table 2.4). These potential revisions can be viewed at: http://www.DSM5.org, and include a change in the title of the disorder to "Generalized Anxiety and Worry Disorder" to better capture its predominant feature. Suggestions for Criterion A include removal of the 6-month criterion and reference to the most common domains of worry. Deletion of DSM-IV's Criterion B (lack of control of worry) is suggested as it has not been shown to have a great effect on identified cases. The revised Criterion B mandates that symptoms be present for 3 months, more days than not (formerly 6 months). This may increase prevalence, but it is hoped that it will identify clinically significant cases who have similar correlates to DSM-IV syndromal cases. In the proposed Criterion C, only 1 symptom is required as there is little evidence to support requiring the 3 symptoms in DSM-IV. The proposed Criterion D introduces a behavioural component and an avoidant criteria. Criterion E (formerly DSM-IV Criterion D) may change the phrasing from "features" to "symptoms", however,

Table 2.4 Proposed Changes for DSM-V

A. Excessive anxiety and worry (apprehensive expectation) about two (or more) domains of activities or events (for example, domains like family, health, finances, and school/work difficulties)

B. The excessive anxiety and worry occur on more days than not for three months or more

C. The anxiety and worry are associated with one or more of the following symptoms:*

1. Restlessness or feeling keyed up or on edge
2. Being easily fatigued
3. Difficulty concentrating or mind going blank
4. Irritability
5. Muscle tension
6. Sleep disturbance (difficulty falling or staying asleep, or restless unsatisfying sleep).

D. The anxiety and worry are associated with one or more of the following behaviours:

a. Marked avoidance of situations in which a negative outcome could occur
b. Marked time and effort preparing for situations in which a negative outcome could occur
c. Marked procrastination in behaviour or decision-making due to worries
d. Repeatedly seeking reassurance due to worries.

E. The focus of the anxiety and worry are not restricted to symptoms of another disorder, such as:

- Panic disorder (e.g., anxiety about having a panic attack)
- Social anxiety disorder (e.g., being embarrassed in public)
- Obsessive-compulsive disorder (e.g., anxiety about being contaminated)
- Separation anxiety disorder (e.g., anxiety about being away from home or close relatives)
- Anorexia nervosa (e.g., fear of gaining weight)
- Somatization disorder (e.g., anxiety about multiple physical complaints)
- Body dysmorphic disorder (e.g., worry about perceived appearance flaws)
- Hypochondriasis (e.g., belief about having a serious illness), and the anxiety and worry do not occur exclusively during post-traumatic stress disorder.**

F. The anxiety, worry, or physical symptoms cause clinically significant distress or impairment in social, occupational, or other important areas of functioning. **

G. The disturbance is not due to the direct physiological effects of a substance (e.g., a drug of abuse, a medication) or a general medical condition (e.g., hyperthyroidism) and does not occur exclusively during a mood disorder, a psychotic disorder, or an autism spectrum disorder.**

* The field trial will include the DSM-IV list of six symptoms to re-evaluate the utility of each one.
** An option that will be tested in the field trial is the possibility of deleting criteria E, F, and G. (from http://www.dsm5.org/ProposedRevisions/Pages/proposedrevision.aspx?rid=167; accessed January 17, 2011)

Criteria E, F (formerly E) and G (formerly F) may be deleted from DSM-V. In addition to the DSM-5 website, Andrews and colleagues (2010) have summarized other options and rationale for potential revisions to the diagnostic classification of GAD.

Whatever ultimately occurs with the classification of GAD in DSM-V, the architects of this new diagnostic system will likely take into account the dimensional nature of anxiety and mood disorders.

2.2 Epidemiology

The prevalence of GAD has been examined worldwide and a broad range of rates have been reported (Table 2.5). The variability between countries can largely be explained by the diagnostic criteria employed (i.e. DSM-III vs. DSM-III-R vs. ICD-10, etc.). In general, Asian countries appear to have much lower prevalence rates of GAD than those in European or North American countries. Lower rates of many psychiatric disorders have been consistently found in Asian populations. This may be due in part to a lack of symptom reporting; however, this likely does not completely account for the variance observed in prevalence.

The US National Comorbidity Survey Replication (NCS-R) was a general population survey in which 9,282 adults aged 18 yrs or older in US households were interviewed between 2001 and 2003; the results of this investigation are considered to be the gold standard in North American psychiatric epidemiology. In this study, 5.7% of respondents met criteria for lifetime DSM-IV GAD, and 3.1% met criteria in the past year (Kessler, Berglund *et al.* 2005; Kessler, Chiu *et al.* 2005).

Data from European studies are relatively consistent with that from the US NCS-R survey. Based on combined data from 27 studies conducted in Europe, it has been estimated that the median 1-yr prevalence of GAD (DSM-IV) is 1.7% and that at least 5.9 million adults in the European Union will have been affected by GAD in the past year (Wittchen and Jacobi 2005). In a review of European studies, the lifetime prevalence of GAD (DSM-IIIR, DSM-IV, ICD-10) ranged from 0.1% to 6.9% (Lieb *et al.* 2005).

GAD is a highly prevalent psychiatric disorder that affects individuals on virtually every continent on the globe. The rates of GAD are highly influenced by diagnostic criteria, however indicating a need for a consistent diagnostic classification system used to determine the true worldwide prevalence.

Table 2.5 Epidemiology of GAD				
Author/year	Criteria	Prevalence 12 month	Prevalence lifetime	Country
Angst et al. (1982)	DSM-III	3.8%	—	Switzerland
Breslau et al. (1985)	DSM-III	11.5% (6 month)**	45%	USA
Favarelli et al. (1989) (same sample)	DSM-III DSM-III-R	— —	5.4% 3.9%	Italy
Blazer et al. (1991)	DSM-III	2.0%–3.6% (three samples)	4.1%–6.6% (three samples)	USA
Chen et al. (1993)	DSM-III	—	7.8% (M) 11.1% (F)	Hong Kong
Wittchen et al. (1994)	DSM-III-R ICD-10	2.0% (M) 4.3% (F) 3.1% (T) 5.0%	3.6% (M) 6.6% (F) 5.1% (T) 8.9%	USA
Offord et al. (1996)	DSM-III-R	0.9% (M) 1.2% (F) 1.1% (T)	—	Canada (ONT)
Bijl et al. (1998)	DSM-III-R	0.8% (M) 1.6% (F)	1.5% (M) 2.9% (F)	Netherlands
Fones et al. (1998)	ICD-10	1.5%	—	Singapore
Ansseau and Rogers (1999)	DSM-IV	—	1.8%	Belgium
Kessler et al. (1999)	DSM-III-R	3.1%–3.3% (two samples)	—	USA
Szadoczky et al. (2000)	DSM-III-R	2.1%	4.6%	Hungary
Carter et al. (2001)	DSM-IV	1.5%	—	Germany
Kringten et al. (2001)	DSM-III-R	1.9%	4.5%	Norway
Kessler et al. (2002)	DSM-III-R	1.0% 1.2% 2.6% 2.9%	2.5% 1.9% 5.3% 5.0%	Brazil Canada Netherlands USA
McConnel et al. (2002)	ICD-10	0.15%	—	Ireland

Table 2.5 (Contd.)				
Author/year	Criteria	Prevalence 12 month	Prevalence lifetime	Country
Hunt et al. (2002)	DSM-IV	3.1%–3.6%	—	Australia
Favarelli et al. (2004)	DSM-IV	2.2% (M) 4.6% (F) 3.5% (T)	—	Italy
Kawakami et al. (2004)	DSM-III-R	0.8% (6 months)	1.4%	Japan
Kessler et al. (2005[a,b])	DSM-IV	3.1%	5.7%	USA
Grant et al. (2005)	DSM-IV	2.1%	4.1%	USA
Lim et al. (2005)	DSM-IV	—	1.5% (M) 4.4% (F) 3.3% (T)	Singapore
Cho et al. (2007)	DSM-IV	0.7% (M) 1.4% (F) 1.0% (T)	1.2% (M) 3.4% (M) 2.3% (T)	Korea
Lee et al. (2007)	DSM-IV	3.4% (M) (6 months)** 4.8% (F) 4.1% (T)	—	Hong Kong

M = Male; F = Female; T = Total; All prevalence rates are total unless otherwise specified; **Some studies give 6-month and not 12-month duration.

References

Amercian Psychiatric Association. (1987). *Diagnostic and Statistical Manual of Mental Disorders: Third Edition, Revised.* American Psychiatric Association, Washington DC.

American Pshychiatric Association. (1994). *Diagnostic and Statistical Manual of Mental Disorders: Fourth Edition.* American Psychiatric Association, Washington DC.

American Psychiatric Association. (2000). *Diagnostic and Statistical Manual of Mental Disorders: Fourth Edition, Text Revision.* American Psychiatric Association, Washington DC.

Andrews G, Anderson TM, Slade T, Suderland M. (2008). Classification of anxiety and depressive disorders: problems and solutions. *Depress Anx*, **25**, 274–81.

Andrews G, Hobbs M, Borkovec TD et al. (2010). Generalized worry disorder: a review of DSM-IV generalized anxiety disorder and options for DSM-V. *Depression & Anxiety*, **27**, 134–47.

[a]Kessler RC, Berglund P, Demler O, Jin R, Merikangas KR, Walters EE. (2005). Lifetime prevalence and age-of-onset distributions of DSM-IV disorders in the national comorbidity survey replication. *Arch Gen Psych*, **62**, 593–603.

[b]Kessler RC, Chiu WT, Demler O, Walters EE. (2005). Prevalence, severity, and comorbidity of 12-month DSM-IV disorders in the national comorbidity survey replication. *Arch Gen Psych*, **62**, 617–27.

Klein DF, Klein HM. (1990). Clinical validation of anxiety syndromes, in: Sartorius N (Ed). *Anxiety: Psychobiological and Clinical Perspectives*. Hemisphere Publishing Corporation, Washington DC, pp. 127–37.

Lieb R, Becker E, Altamura C. (2005). The epidemiology of generalized anxiety disorder in Europe. *Eur Neuropsychopharmacol*, **15**, 445–42.

Marten PA, Brown TA, Barlow DH, Borkovec TD, Shear MK, Lydiard RB. (1993) Evaluation of the ratings comprising the associated symptom criterion of DSM-III-R generalized anxiety disorder. *J Nerv Mental Dis*, **181**, 676–82.

Mennin DS, Heimberg RG, Fresco DM, Ritter MR. (2008). Is generalized anxiety disorder an anxiety or mood disorder? Considering multiple factors as we ponder the fate of GAD. *Depress Anx*, **25**, 289–99.

Rickels K, Rynn MA. (2001). What is generalized anxiety disorder? *J Clin Psychiat*, **62** (Suppl 11), 4–12.

Slade T, Andrews G. (2001). DSM-IV and ICD-10 generalized anxiety disorder: discrepant diagnosis and associated disability. *Soc Psychiatr Psychiatric Epidemiol*, **36**, 45–51.

Wittchen HU, Jacobi F. (2005). Size and burden of mental disorders in Europe—a critical review and apraisal of 27 studies. *Eur Neuropsychopharmacol*, **15**, 357–36.

World Health Organization. (1992). *The ICD-10 Classification of Mental and Behavioural Disorders: Clinical Descriptions and Diagnostic Guidelines*. WHO, Geneva.

Chapter 3

Clinical features

Beth Patterson, Michael Van Ameringen, and Mark H. Pollack

Key points

- Only a third to a half of generalized anxiety disorder (GAD) cases receive a proper diagnosis due to its somatic presentation.
- GAD afflicts twice as many women than men, has a later age of onset with the highest rates found in the 45 to 59 age group.
- The course of GAD is typically chronic with episodes lasting between 6½ and 10 yrs, and sometimes longer
- GAD usually presents with co-morbid psychiatric conditions often posing a diagnostic challenge.

3.1 Presentation

Generalized anxiety disorder (GAD) is one of the most common anxiety disorders seen in adults in general, and is even more prevalent in the general medical setting. It is frequently misdiagnosed or overlooked as patients often present with predominantly somatic rather than cognitive or psychological symptoms. Common presenting physical complaints include:

- Insomnia
- Muscle tension, trembling, twitching, aching, soreness
- Cold, clammy hands
- Dry mouth
- Sweating
- Nausea or diarrhoea
- Urinary frequency
- Tachycardia, palpitations
- Dizziness, light-headedness
- Breathing difficulties
- Numbness, tingling
- Hot or cold flushes.

The aetiology of these physical or somatic symptoms may remain unexplained following medical evaluation, and contribute to the observation that patients with GAD are over-represented among high utilizers of health care. Physical symptoms can be the main avenue through which GAD patients express their distress (known as somatization) and clinicians are therefore often obliged to search for underlying physical pathology in patients who may be reluctant to accept that they are suffering from a psychiatric illness. In a large German study in a primary care population, only 13% of patients with GAD described anxiety as their primary complaint. Half the patients with GAD presented with somatic (medical) illnesses or complaints of pain and sleep disturbance (Kessler and Wittchen 2002).

GAD is so often disguised by physical complaints that only 33% to 53% of GAD cases receive a proper diagnosis. In contrast, upwards of 95% of patients are correctly diagnosed if the presenting complaint is anxiety or depression.

Patients with GAD experience uncontrollable and excessive worry about day-to-day matters such as finances, family, work, or health. GAD patients often worry about the impact of their worrying. For example, they may be concerned that worry will damage their health or they may think that negative things will occur if they do not worry enough. These individuals report more worry about the future than patients with other anxiety problems. Worry in GAD is uncontrollable, chronic, exaggerated, and impairs functioning. These characteristics seem to differentiate GAD from normal worry. Clinical vignettes of two patients with GAD are provided in Boxes 3.1 and 3.2 below.

Box 3.1 Andy's story

'Andy' was a 42-yr-old, married man who went to see his general practitioner for excessive worrying. His history revealed excessive worry, dating back to his childhood, where he felt jittery and on-guard most of the time while worrying about weather-related events. After age 10, he recalled being keenly aware of his family's financial situation and constantly worried that they would not have enough money. As a student, he worried about his academic performance but would procrastinate, as the task of completing assignments, or studying seemed overwhelming. Prior to seeing his physician, Andy's worrying had increased significantly to the point where it was difficult to control. He had been excessively worried about his performance on the job (despite good performance reviews) and often felt overwhelmed. The worry became so intense, that he had resigned 1 yr prior to his current presentation to 'take time off and try to settle down'. He was surprised to discover that his

Box 3.1 (Contd.)

worry did not abate with the absence of the job stressor. The content of his current worries include completing household chores, feeling like he never had enough time to get things done, the safety and health of his young daughter and wife as well as his own health and that of every member of his extended family. His family physician had recently prescribed a cholesterol-lowering agent, but Andy had not started this medication as he was afraid of potential side effects and was avoiding having his cholesterol level checked. Andy avoided watching television news reports as stories concerning natural disasters, crimes, and wars would induce thoughts and images which were difficult for him to let go of. His financial worries were so intense that he often avoided looking at his finances. He also reported intense worry about the future and although he had two employment opportunities lined up, he could not deal with the uncertainty of not having his future mapped out completely. Despite obtaining an undergraduate university degree, Andy had a history of working at low-level jobs and staying at them for long periods of time. He reported fearing change and doubted his abilities. Andy described feeling restless and on edge most of the time, he also experienced muscle tension, irritability, difficulty concentrating, and often had trouble sleeping. He recognized his worry as excessive but felt powerless to stop it. Andy had no significant medical history, no prior psychiatric history, and did not take any medications on a regular basis.

Box 3.2 Grace's story

'Grace' was a 55-yr-old, unemployed, divorced woman who was referred for assessment and treatment of excessive worry and anxiety by her gastroenterologist. Grace reported feeling anxious since the age of six. In childhood, she worried about choking on her food, death, her school work and about the safety of her parents. Grace endorsed a marked increase in her worry over the past 7 yrs after her three children had moved out of the house. She described excessive and uncontrollable day-to-day worries about her future, family, friends, and finances. When she was working she constantly worried about doing a good job and pleasing her employer. She reported significant worries about her health and ongoing stomach problems (which included frequent episodes of abdominal pain, gas,

Box 3.2 *(Contd.)*

and diarrhoea). Each episode of abdominal pain or diarrhoea would be followed by intense worry that she had a serious illness which was likely fatal (usually stomach cancer). This worry persisted despite her understanding of the relationship between her gastrointestinal symptoms and her anxiety and despite numerous medical investigations with negative findings. As a result of these symptoms, Grace had quit her job as a supervisor at a donut shop 6 months prior to being seen. Grace also worried that the elevator in her apartment building would break down and that she might faint while having a shower and that no one would know. Other daily worries included that she would some day be a burden on her children and have no money to pay for her own funeral. Associated with her excessive worrying were feelings of inattention, restlessness, and fatigue. She reported tension in her shoulders, poor concentration, initial and mid-insomnia, being easily startled, poor appetite with fluctuations in her weight. Additional symptoms included frequent urination, bouts of diarrhoea, dry mouth, decreased motivation, and poor self-care during periods of intense worry. She found that her worry would intensify at night. According to Grace, she had significant anticipatory anxiety so that one worry would lead to another to the point where her thoughts are racing. She acknowledged that her worrying was excessive and markedly interfered in her life.

3.2 **Age of onset**

Unlike most anxiety disorders, GAD has a later age of onset and its prevalence seems to increase with age, with the highest rates found in those aged 45 to 59 yrs. GAD seems to develop somewhere between late teens and late 20s. Very few prevalence studies have involved individuals over the age of 65 yrs; however, there are indications that elderly individuals in the general population continue to have high rates of GAD. A large epidemiological study in Germany (Carter *et al.* 2001) found only a handful of respondents who were younger than 25 yrs, met full criteria for DSM-IV GAD. Data from the National Comorbidity Survey—Replication (NCS-R) indicated that GAD prevalence increases from young adulthood (4.1%) to a peak in middle adulthood (6.8% to 7.7%) and a decline in rates for those over 60 yrs of age (3.6%) (Kessler *et al.* 2005). Moreover, GAD in older adults appears to be more chronic and the duration of episodes of worry are longer when compared to younger adults. Among the 7,200 adults who reported at least 3 months of worrying in the German National Health Interview and Examination Survey Study, subjects aged 35 to 65 yrs were more likely than subjects aged 18 to 34 yrs to report a duration of 6 months of worrying (Carter *et al.* 2001).

3.3 Gender and socio-demographic correlates

Epidemiological reports across multiple countries have found the rate of GAD among women to be roughly double that for men. In people aged over 35 yrs, rates of GAD have been shown to be upwards of three times more prevalent in women than in men. In the original NCS, the lifetime prevalence of GAD increased steadily in women after their mid-20s and by the age of 45 yrs, 1 in 10 women surveyed had reported a history of GAD. GAD appears to be more common among people who are unmarried, widowed, separated, or divorced, of low socioeconomic status, and among those unemployed or not working (i.e. homemakers). The NCS found no significant associations between urbanicity, income, education, and religion. Some reports have indicated that those who are part of racial minority groups have higher indices of GAD; however in others, racial minorities have reported lower rates of GAD than Caucasians. In a recent study African-American subjects with GAD reported a greater positive affect than Caucasians subjects; however, no significant differences were found in terms of the prevalence of GAD, nor on measures of symptom severity (Brenes *et al.* 2008).

There is a dearth of information concerning cross-cultural differences in the presentation of GAD. Cross-cultural studies of depression have shown that there is a greater somatic focus in Asian cultures (including Taiwanese, Chinese, Vietnamese, Indian, Filipino, and Hong Kong populations) relative to Western cultures. Currently there is only one published report concerning cross-cultural differences in GAD (Hoge *et al.* 2006), which examined Nepali versus American subjects with GAD. Although no significant differences were found in symptom severity, subjects in Nepal had higher somatic sub-scale scores compared to American subjects who had higher psychological subscale scores. This phenomenon has been conceptualized in the literature in a number of ways. It may be that a difference exists between core ideologies in Western and Asian medicine as traditional Asian medicine does not distinguish between mind and body. This lack of distinction would render separation of anxiety symptom type irrelevant in Asian cultures as well as increasing the probability that psychological distress will manifest as somatic symptomatology. It has also been suggested that the semantic framework for expressing affect differs between Western and Asian cultures such that Asian cultures are less inclined towards intense introspection of personal affective states making some emotions difficult to articulate. Given that a focus on somatic presentation of psychological distress has been seen across a broad scope of cultures, some researchers have argued that it is in fact the global norm and that the Western tendency towards 'psychologization' warrants examination and explanation.

3.4 Course and prognosis

The course of GAD is typically chronic. Symptoms of GAD tend to wax and wane over time, with episodes lasting between 6½ and 10 yrs, and sometimes longer. Episodes or relapses are commonly triggered by stress and seem to be more persistent as people age. Long-term studies have revealed low rates of remission (less than one-third of patients spontaneously remit) even in individuals who have received treatment.

The presence of other psychiatric disorders is related to a poorer prognosis in GAD. Co-morbid alcohol or other substance use disorders, significantly decreases the likelihood of recovery from GAD and significantly increases the likelihood of GAD recurrence (Bruce *et al.* 2005).

Some of the most comprehensive longitudinal data have come from the Harvard/Brown Anxiety Research Program. It was a prospective observational longitudinal study including 167 participants with DSM III-R GAD who were followed for 5 yrs. At 5-yr follow-up, 38% had achieved full remission (occasional or no symptoms for at least eight consecutive weeks) and 47% had achieved partial remission (reduction in symptoms for at least 8 weeks). At 3-yr follow-up, 27% of those who had reached full remission experienced relapse in their symptoms. Thirty-nine per cent of those who had reached partial remission relapsed. The presence of co-morbidity or chronicity did not inhibit development of remission. Full or partial remissions were less likely to occur in patients with poor relationships and personality disorders. This study also revealed that participants were more likely to be taking an antidepressant if they also had one or more co-morbid conditions.

3.5 Psychiatric co-morbidity

It is rare to see individuals present with GAD without co-morbidity. Although there is considerable variation in the literature, a high proportion of individuals (up to 98%) with GAD report co-morbid anxiety disorders (agoraphobia, panic disorder, simple phobia, social phobia), mood disorders (dysthymia, major depressive disorder, mania), or substance use disorders (substance abuse or dependence). Major depression, social phobia, and specific phobia are most common however, panic disorder, agoraphobia, and post-traumatic stress disorder (PTSD) are also frequently encountered in GAD patients (Table 3.1). Prevalence rates of attention deficit hyperactivity disorder (ADHD) amongst individuals with GAD range between 10% and 45%; however, little is known about the relationship between these two disorders. Some authors have speculated that the high rates of co-morbidity are a result of a diagnostic artifact in adults with ADHD along with symptoms of reduced stress tolerance. Vesga-López and colleagues (2008) found gender differences in GAD comorbidity using data from the National Epidemiology Survey on Alcohol and Related Conditions (NESARC). Men with GAD reported significantly higher rates of comorbid alcohol and substance use disorders, nicotine dependence and antisocial personality disorder. Women with GAD had significantly higher prevalence of comorbid mood disorders (with the exception of bipolar), and anxiety disorders (with the exception of social anxiety disorder).

Studies in children and adolescents support the findings in adults of high rates of co-morbidity in individuals with GAD. Earlier studies using the diagnosis of 'over-anxious disorder' (from DSM-III-R) have

Table 3.1 Prevalence of DSM-III-R disorders co-morbid with GAD		
DSM-IV Disorder	**1-month prevalence (%)**	**Lifetime prevalence (%)**
Mania	12.1	10.5
Major depression	38.6	62.5
Dysthymia	22.1	39.5
Panic disorder	22.6	23.5
Agoraphobia	26.7	25.7
Simple phobia	24.5	35.1
Social phobia	23.2	34.4
Alcohol abuse/dependence	11.2	37.6
Drug abuse/dependence	5.1	27.6
Any of the above disorders	66.3	90.4
Data from National Comorbidity Survey (Wittchen et al. 1994).		

shown rates of co-morbidity in children as high as 96%. The most common co-morbid conditions in childhood seem to be separation anxiety disorder, social phobia, and depressive disorders. There also appears to be a strong association between over-anxious disorder and major depressive disorder (MDD). In children and adolescents with ADHD, GAD is one of the most prevalent co-morbid anxiety disorders (as high as 12.8%). One study found particular association between females with the combined subtype of ADHD (hyperactivity/impulsivity plus inattention) and higher rates of GAD.

In the elderly, co-morbidity is also high with only a small minority having only pure GAD. By far, the most common co-morbid condition seen in the elderly is MDD (55% to 91%) in studies of nursing home and community populations.

3.6 **Order of onset**

The literature concerning which disorder comes first—GAD or a co-morbid psychiatric condition—is equivocal. In a combined analysis of four large-scale epidemiological studies, GAD preceded the development of another anxiety disorder in 25% of cases and preceded the development of a mood disorder in 21% of cases (Kessler et al. 2002). These results were supported by another study which found that GAD preceded the onset of panic disorder (52% of cases), panic disorder with agoraphobia (72% of cases), PTSD (70% of cases), and MDD (70% of cases). The presence of GAD was found to be a significant predictor of MDD in both 12-month and lifetime analyses. This relationship was stronger than any other disorder pair examined. A diagnosis of GAD was found to predict an increased rate of onset of MDD >10 yrs after the initial GAD diagnosis (Rodriguez et al. 2004). However, in a prospective longitudinal study GAD onset occurred first in only a third of individuals while major depression onset occurred first in a third of individuals and major depression and GAD began concurrently in a third of participants (Moffitt et al. 2007). Although the evidence supporting a strong relationship between these disorders is clear, assertions regarding order of onset remain uncertain.

3.7 **Heritability**

Though MDD and GAD heritability patterns are very similar, some twin studies have revealed that environmental determinants for GAD and MDD are distinct. As well, socio-demographic predictors also differ for both disorders. This suggests that although MDD and GAD may come from similar genetic origins, they remain dissociable based on environmental and social factors (see Chapter 4 for more details).

3.8 **Differentiating between GAD and co-morbid psychiatric conditions**

The relationship between MDD and GAD is important not only to address in terms of the potential re-classification of the disorders as previously discussed, but also it may have therapeutic implications (for instance whether benzodiazepine monotherapy may be an appropriate option) in some patients for practitioners attempting to distinguish between the two. There is significant symptom overlap between MDD and GAD. As previously described, a DSM-IV-TR diagnosis of GAD is based upon the presence of excessive, uncontrollable worry plus at least three of six associated symptoms. Four of these six symptoms are also characteristics of MDD (restlessness, fatigue, difficulty concentrating, and sleep disturbance). Moreover, many individuals with MDD also report symptoms of anxiety such as worry, apprehension, and irritability. For the clinician, the diagnosis of MDD versus GAD may be solely based upon the presence of anhedonia and/or a depressed mood which are hallmark symptoms of MDD. In instances where an individual would meet criteria for both MDD and GAD, it is important to determine if the generalized anxiety occurs in the absence of episodes of depression.

In order to differentiate between GAD and other anxiety disorders, it is useful to attempt to characterize the worry. In GAD, the worry is excessive, chronic and occurs more days than not. The content of the worry encompasses a wide variety of issues from day-to-day matters to future events, financial issues, social, health, or safety of the individual or of loved ones. Worry can be a feature of other anxiety disorders; however, the content is generally quite different. For example, in panic disorder the worry centres around experiencing physical symptoms associated with panic attacks as well a losing control, dying, or of having another panic attack. In social phobia the worry is focused on being negatively evaluated by others and in PTSD the worry is related to being reminded of a specific event or trauma. In obsessive-compulsive disorder (OCD), the worry is tied in with repetitive obsessions and tends to be centred around issues such as contamination or doubting and are also associated with neutralizing or ritualized compulsive behaviours. Table 3.2 compares GAD worry to that of other psychiatric conditions.

3.9 **Medical co-morbidity**

GAD is strongly associated with somatic conditions including chest pain, chronic fatigue syndrome, irritable bowel syndrome, hypertension, diabetes, heart disease, respiratory problems, and migraine (Table 3.3).

Table 3.2 Differentiating GAD from other psychiatric disorders

GAD	Depression
• Focus of worry is on negative events that have occurred in the past but also those which may occur in the future • Worry is accompanied by anxiety, but not necessarily guilt or feelings of worthlessness	• Focus of worry (described as ruminations) is on negative events that have occurred in the past • Ruminations are usually accompanied by profound feelings of guilt or worthlessness

GAD	OCD
• Content of worries often refer to potentially 'real-life' events and though excessive are not viewed as inappropriate • Worry is cyclical (one worry leads to another)	• Obsessive thoughts are considered intrusive, unwanted, and inappropriate and usually result in significant distress • Same thought or image is repeated

GAD	Panic disorder
• Focus of worries are actual 'real-life' events • Physical symptoms associated with GAD are not usually interpreted as being dangerous in and of themselves	• Focus of worry is the fear of having a panic attack/physical symptoms in situations where previous attacks have occurred or where help/escape are not readily available • Often involves avoidance of situations for fear of having a panic attack (agoraphobia)

GAD	Social anxiety disorder
• Social-interactional worries may be present as one of many day-to-day worries • Social-interactional worries do not usually lead to avoidance	• Focus of the worry is specifically related to social and performance situations where the individual perceives negative evaluation by others • Social and performance situations are usually avoided and cause significant distress and impairment

GAD	Hypochondriasis
• Excessive worry about several topics, including disease or illness • Illness worry concerns potentially contracting a disease in the future, but not the belief that one is already present but undiagnosed • If medical consultation is sought, these patients may respond well (at least transiently) to reassurance	• Excessive preoccupation with one or more diseases or illnesses • Worry that the disease or illness has already been contracted and is undiagnosed • Excessive medical consultations and investigations, however reassurance is ineffective or short-lived • Physical symptoms are mistakenly understood as signs of a serious illness

Table 3.3 Medical conditions with significant associations to GAD

Cardiac problems (includes hypertension, chest pain, stroke, heart disease)	Migraine and tension headaches
Irritable bowel syndrome	Chronic pain conditions (includes neuropathic pain)
Gastrointestinal disease (includes ulcers, hernias)	Dermatological disorders
Respiratory disorders (includes COPD, asthma)	Osteopathic conditions (including osteoporosis, hip, joint, and back problems)
Endocrine disorders (diabetes, thyroid disorders	Chronic fatigue syndrome

Upwards of one-third of respiratory patients have been reported to have an anxiety disorder. Higher rates of respiratory problems have been found in GAD patients and increased rates of GAD have been found in asthma patients. The presence of a co-morbid anxiety disorder with pulmonary disease is associated with a greater use of treatments including the use of steroids and bronchodilators, a poorer quality of life, and an increase in hospitalization (Simon et al. 2006).

Individuals with GAD or panic disorder have been shown to have a 5.9-fold increased risk of cardiac problems (after controlling for gender, depression, and substance abuse). In a large longitudinal study, men with high phobic anxiety had a threefold greater risk of coronary heart disease and a four- to sixfold increase risk of sudden cardiac death as compared to those with low phobic anxiety. In a similar longitudinal study of women, phobic anxiety was associated with fatal coronary heart disease and sudden cardiac death (Albert et al. 2005). In one study, 40% of patients developed clinically significant anxiety and 27% met criteria for GAD following a stroke. In this study, GAD patients had posterior right hemisphere lesions, whereas patients with mild anxiety had lesions in the anterior right hemisphere (Hidalgo and Davidson 2001).

Studies have also examined the association between anxiety disorders and thyroid dysfunction. In the general population, ~2.7% of the population has a history of thyroid disease. In a retrospective study looking at patients entering clinical trials, 10% of GAD patients had a history of thyroid difficulties compared with 2% of panic patients and 4% of the social phobics; only GAD was found to have a significantly higher rate of thyroid abnormalities than the general population (Simon et al. 2002). Women with Graves' disease (with associated hyperthyroidism and ophthalmopathy) were significantly more likely to have GAD than normal controls. Anxiety symptoms predated the onset of Graves' disease in a large proportion of cases (Muller et al. 2005).

In adults with diabetes mellitus, GAD has been found to be the most prevalent co-morbid anxiety disorder. Rates of GAD in diabetic populations (13.5% current; 20.5% lifetime) are much higher than those in the community (Muller *et al.* 2005).

GAD and migraine have been linked in several reports. In epidemiological samples examining migraine sufferers, a lifetime prevalence of GAD was found in 10.2% compared to 1.9% in respondents without migraines (Guillem *et al.* 1999).

3.10 **Differentiating between medical conditions and GAD**

The recognition and diagnosis of GAD is complicated by the fact that it frequently co-exists with other medical or psychiatric conditions. GAD patients often present with somatic (medical) symptoms, which may help to explain why so many sufferers are undiagnosed and untreated, despite frequent visits to their primary care physicians.

It is important for clinicians to be cognizant of the high association between GAD and pulmonary, cardiac, endocrine, and gastrointestinal conditions when treating patients for these medical problems.

3.11 **Suicide risk**

Anxiety disorders are associated with an increased risk of suicidal behaviour. The rates of suicide risk have been reported as ten times higher than the rates in the general population and indicate that anxiety disorder patients, including those with GAD, should be carefully evaluated for suicide risk. Moreover, the presence of a co-morbid mood disorder, especially MDD, appears to significantly increase the risk of suicidal behaviour.

3.12 **Burden of illness**

The burden of illness associated with GAD is broad. It results not just in marked distress to the affected individual, but incurs a great cost to society in terms of both direct costs such as increased healthcare utilization and indirect costs such as lost work productivity. Patients with GAD, with or without co-morbid MDD, have been shown to be high utilizers of healthcare resources when compared with patients unaffected by either disorder. It has been reported that people with GAD (with or without co-morbid MDD) make twice as many visits to primary care physicians as those with neither GAD or MDD. In a German study of primary care, patients with GAD or GAD with co-morbid MDD visited their primary care physician more than once every month. The average frequency of visits to specialists was also higher in people with GAD than among those who had neither GAD nor MDD, with over 40% of patients with GAD and/or MDD also making two or more visits to other specialists (excluding psychiatrists) in the year preceding the study. Interestingly in this study, only around one-quarter of all patients with GAD and MDD had seen a psychiatrist or psychotherapist in the previous year (Wittchen et al. 2002). Consistent with these findings, results from the Australian National Survey of Mental Health and Well-Being found that over half of individuals with GAD had seen a health-care provider, although only 14% of those had seen a mental health specialist (Hunt et al. 2002).

A 1999 US study examined the monetary value of the burden associated with anxiety disorders. The cost to the US economy was $42.3 billion in 1990 (equal to $63.1 billion in 1998 dollars) in terms of psychiatric and non-psychiatric medical treatment, mortality, as well as reductions in work productivity. The largest portion of societal costs was accounted for by the direct costs of non-psychiatric medical treatment (54% of the total), psychiatric treatment (31%), and pharmaceutical costs (2%). Indirect costs (mortality, excess absenteeism, and decreased work productivity) accounted for 13% of the total societal costs (Greenberg et al. 1999). In a prospective, naturalistic, longitudinal study of anxiety disorders in primary care, subjects aged 18 yrs and over were asked at intake to rate how much difficulty they had been having with their normal activities or tasks, both inside and outside the house, because of their physical and emotional health, during the preceding 4 weeks (Maki et al. 2003). Over 50% of GAD patients reported having at least some difficulty with their usual activities in the previous 4 weeks. Nearly one-third of the patients had 'much difficulty' with their normal activities, and 2% were completely incapacitated because of their physical and emotional health.

The Midlife Development in the United States survey (MIDUS) involved a nationally representative sample of 3,032 non-institutionalized individuals aged 25 to 74 yrs (Kessler et al. 2001). In this study, individuals with GAD reported greater functional impairment than individuals with other chronic and disabling medical conditions, including arthritis and asthma (Figure 3.1). On average, GAD sufferers were severely disabled (i.e. could not work or function normally) for 10 days in the previous month. Of the 29 physical and mental illnesses analysed in this study, GAD was associated with the highest risk of work impairment. At least 1 day of lost or reduced work was reported by 61% of patients with GAD, compared with 39% of patients with arthritis, 45% of patients with asthma, and 40% of patients with diabetes.

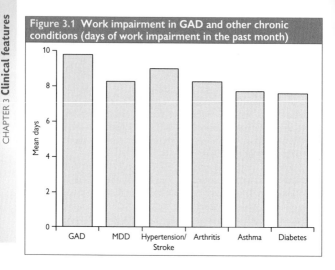

Figure 3.1 Work impairment in GAD and other chronic conditions (days of work impairment in the past month)

Results from a similar community-based survey of 4,181 individuals in Germany support these findings indicating that GAD is associated with a considerable burden of lost productivity. In this study, over half of the respondents with GAD reported work loss and/or impairment in the past month. The proportion of subjects with GAD who reported work loss/impairment exceeded that observed in those with pure MDD. Having both GAD and MDD was associated with the greatest work impairment/loss as well as the greatest average number of lost workdays in the past month. Only 5% of respondents who did not have GAD or MDD reported work loss/impairment in the past month (Wittchen *et al.* 2000). This study also examined functional impairment and found that individuals with GAD scored significantly lower on quality of life measures especially in the domains of general health, mental health, and vitality than those without GAD.

3.13 Summary

GAD represents a significant burden to afflicted individuals, to their employers, and to the health-care system. Individuals with GAD often seek treatment but are misdiagnosed due to the high degree of somatization and co-morbidity associated with the disorder. These people may 'slip through the cracks' or continue to receive fruitless medical workups or endure marked distress and disability without appropriate diagnosis and targeted treatment of the anxiety. When an individual presents with excessive or uncontrollable anxiety or worry, it is certainly important to consider potential alterative causes of the symptoms such as medical or other psychiatric conditions. However, given that patients with GAD frequently have co-morbid conditions and that anxiety disorders are more common in patients with certain medical and psychiatric conditions, the diagnosis of other disorders should not preclude the diagnosis of GAD, nor the converse.

References

Albert CM, Chae CU, Rexrode KM, Manson JE, Kawachi I. (2005). Phobic anxiety and risk of coronary heart disease and sudden cardiac death among women. *Circulation*, **111**, 480–87.

Brenes GA, Knudson M, McCall V, Williamson JD, Miller ME, Stanley MA. (2008). Age and racial differences in the presentation and treatment of generalized anxiety disorder in primary care. *J Anx Dis*, **22**, 1128–34.

Bruce SE, Yonkers KA, Otto MW et al. (2005). Influence of psychiatric comorbidity on recovery and recurrence in generalized anxiety disorder, social phobia, and panic disorder: a 12-year study. *Am J Psych*, **162**, 1179–87.

Carter RM, Wittchen HU, Pfister H, Kessler RC. (2001). One year prevalence of sub threshold and threshold DSM-IV generalized anxiety disorder in a nationally representative sample. *Depress Anx*, **13**, 78–88.

Greenberg PE, Sisitsky T, Kessler RC et al. (1999). The economic burden of anxiety disorders in the 1990s. *J Clin Psych*, **60**, 427–35.

Guillem E, Pelissolo A, Lepine JP. (2009). Mental disorders and migraine: epidemiologic studies. *Encephale*, **25**, 436–42.

Hidalgo RB, Davidson JRT. (2001). Generalized anxiety disorder: an important clinical concern. *Med Clin North Am*, **83**, 691–710.

Hoge EA, Tamrakar SM, Christian KM et al. (2006). Cross-cultural differences in somatic presentation in patients with generalized anxiety disorder. *J Nerv Mental Dis*, **194**, 962–6.

Hunt C, Issakidis C, Andrews G. (2002). DSM-IV generalized anxiety disorder in the Australian National Survey of Mental Health and Well-Being. *Psychol Med*, **32**, 649–59.

Kessler RC, Andrade LH, Bijl RV, Offard DR, Demler OV, Stein DJ. (2002). The effects of co-morbidity on the onset and persistence of generalized anxiety disorder in the ICPE surveys. *Psychol Med*, **32**, 1213–25.

Kessler RC, Berglund P, Demler O, Jin R, Merikangas KR, Walters EE. (2005). Lifetime prevalence and age-of-onset distributions of DSM-IV disorders in the National Comorbidity Survey Replication. *Arch Gen Psych*, **62**, 593–603.

Kessler RC, Mickelson KD, Barber C, Wang P. (2001). The association between chronic and medical conditions and work impairment. In: Rossi AC (ed.) *Caring and doing for others: Social Responsibility in the do-*

mains of Family, Work and Community. University of Chicago Press, Chicago, IL. Ch. 10, pp.403–27.

Kessler RC, Wittchen HU. (2002). Patterns and correlates of generalized anxiety disorder in community samples. *J Clin Psych*, **63** (Suppl 8), 4–10.

Maki K, Weisberg RS, Keller MB, Spencer MJ, Culpepper L. (2003). Psychosocial and Work Impairment in Primary Care Patients with GAD. Poster presented at the 156th Annual Meeting of the American Psychiatric Association, March 20–23. Toronto, Ontario, Canada.

Moffitt TE, Harrington HL, Caspi A et al. (2007). Cumulative and sequential comorbidity in a birth cohort followed prospectively to age 32 years. *Arch Gen Psych*, **64**, 651–60.

Muller JE, Koen L, Stein DJ. (2005). Anxiety and medical disorders. *Curr Psych Rep*, **7**, 245–51.

Rodriguez BF, Weisberg RB, Pagano ME, Machan JT, Culpepper L, Keller MB. (2004). Frequency and patterns of psychiatric comorbidity in a sample of primary care patients with anxiety disorders. *Compr Psych*, **45**, 129–37.

Simon NM, Blacker D, Korbly NB et al. (2002). Hypothyroidism and hyperthyroidism in anxiety disorders revisited: new data and literature review. *J Affect Disord*, **69**, 209–17.

Simon NM, Weiss AM, Kradin R et al. (2006). The relationship of anxiety disorders, anxiety sensitivity and pulmonary dysfunction with dyspnea-related distress and avoidance. *J Nerv Mental Dis*, **194**, 951–7.

Vesga-López O, Schneier FR, Wang S et al. (2008). Gender differences in generalized anxiety disorder: results from the National Epidemiological Survey on Alcohol and Related Conditions (NESARC). *J Clin Psychiatry* **69**, 1606–16.

Wittchen HU, Carter RM, Pfister H, Montgomery SA, Kessler RC. (2000). Disabilities and quality of life in pure and comorbid generalized anxiety disorder and major depression in a national survey. *Int Clin Psychopharmacol*, **15**, 319–28.

Wittchen HU, Kessler RC, Beesdo K, Krause P, Höfler M, Hoyer J. (2002). Generalized anxiety and depression in primary care: prevalence, recognition, and management. *J Clin Psych*, **63** (Suppl 8), 24–34.

Wittchen HU, Zhao S, Kessler RC, Eaton WW. (1994). DSM-III-R generalized anxiety disorder in the National Comorbidity Survey. *Arch Gen Psych* **51**, 355–64.

Chapter 4

Neurobiology

Catherine Mancini, Michael Van Ameringen, Beth Patterson, and Mark H. Pollack

> ### Key points
> - The study of neurobiology in generalized anxiety disorder (GAD) is in its infancy.
> - Key neurological structures thought to be involved in GAD include the amygdala and insula.

4.1 Introduction

Our understanding of the underlying pathogenesis of generalized anxiety disorder (GAD) is still evolving. There have been few neurobiological studies specific to GAD, and much of this literature examines the neurobiology of GAD in terms of conceptual frameworks rather than evidence relating to specific functional or anatomical abnormalities.

4.2 Neuroimaging

Neuroimaging studies in anxiety disorders have provided researchers with evidence that several neurological structures are involved in anxiety and fear response. The amygdala is a structure located in the limbic system and has been implicated in fear-processing in terms of mediating fear response and fear conditioning. It is thought to exhibit hyperactivity in response to threat-related stimuli (Figure 4.1). The medial prefrontal cortex (mPFC) is involved in emotion regulation and exerts cortical influence on the amygdala. It is thought that fear-conditioned responses are perpetuated by deficiencies in the extinguishing of these responses by the mPFC. Other neurological structures thought to play a role in anxiety disorders include the anterior cingulate cortex (ACC) (attention to emotional stimuli), medial prefrontal gyrus (mPFG), insula (interoception and visceral response), hippocampus and posterior cingulate cortex (PCC) (explicit and contextual memory) (Britton and Rauch 2008). The main structures of the limbic system are shown in Figures 4.2 and 4.3.

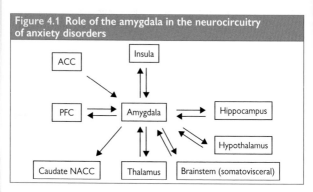

Figure 4.1 Role of the amygdala in the neurocircuitry of anxiety disorders

Neuroimaging studies in GAD are at a very preliminary stage and information implicating specific central nervous system (CNS) structures is relatively scant. Studies using DSM-III and III-R definitions of GAD have indicated altered functioning in the following areas:

- Decreased occipital lobe metabolism following benzodiazepine administration
- High metabolic rates in parts of the occipital, temporal, and frontal lobe metabolism and cerebellum relative to normal controls
- Temporal lobe abnormalities
- Increased activity in frontal regions
- Decrease in basal ganglia metabolism which is reversed with treatment
- Decreased density of benzodiazepine receptors in left temporal pole.

More recently, a functional magnetic resonance imaging (fMRI) study in adolescents with DSM-IV GAD demonstrated a bias away from angry faces and a greater ventrolateral prefrontal cortex activation during an attention task. Amygdala activation was not detected in this study, a finding contrary to that of most anxiety disorders (Monk et al. 2006). However, in a study which compared children with GAD or panic disorder (PD) to healthy controls, exaggerated amygdala activation in response to fearful faces was found (Thomas et al. 2001). In another study using fMRI, adolescents with and without GAD were asked how afraid they felt while viewing fearful versus happy faces. Individuals with GAD (N=15) showed increased activation in the ventral prefrontal cortex, in the anterior cingulate cortex (an area involved in self-reflection) and amygdala as compared to controls (N=20) (McClure et al., 2007). Paulesu and colleagues (2010) recently published an fMRI study of 8 adults with DSM-IV GAD, compared to 12 normal controls. Activation of the anterior cingulate and dorsal medial prefrontal cortex was seen in both GAD patients and controls during worry paradigms. However, unlike controls, individuals with GAD showed persistent activation of these areas during resting state and empathy paradigms for sad faces. The authors concluded that dysregulation in the medial prefrontal and anterior cingulate regions may underpin the inability to stop worrying in GAD.

The insula is a CNS structure which has been shown to be key in processing information about physiological state including changes in heart rate, galvanic skin response, and vagus nerve activity. In adult populations, altered insula activation has been shown in GAD patients following effective treatment with citalopram (Willour *et al.* 2004). In a fMRI study using affective stimuli (wall of faces), it was found that

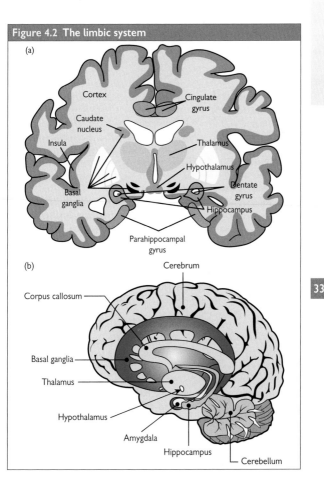

Figure 4.2 The limbic system

(a)

Cortex

Cingulate gyrus

Caudate nucleus

Insula

Thalamus

Hypothalamus

Basal ganglia

Dentate gyrus

Hippocampus

Parahippocampal gyrus

(b)

Cerebrum

Corpus callosum

Basal ganglia

Thalamus

Hypothalamus

Amygdala

Hippocampus

Cerebellum

bilateral insula activation in response to an ambiguous stimulus was related to the degree to which uncertainty is processed as being aversive. The insula may function as a prediction signal, indicating the possibility of future aversive interoception (Simmons *et al.* 2008).

4.3 Neurobiology

4.3.1 Key neurochemical systems involved in GAD

A number of neurochemical systems have been implicated in anxiety and fear response, though the precise nature of their association with GAD remains uncertain.

4.3.2 Corticotropin-releasing hormone (CRH)

There is some evidence to suggest that the neuropeptide CRH may play a role in GAD. CRH is produced in the hypothalamus but is widely distributed throughout the brain. CRH serves as a neurotransmitter in the stress response and the adaptation of emotional behaviour. It is mediated by two main receptors: CRH-1 and CRH-2, which are distributed in brain regions including the locus ceruleus, paraventricular nucleus (PVN), amygdala, hippocampus, and cerebral cortex.

In a study by Tafet and colleagues (2001) in which cortisol levels were monitored in GAD and major depressive disorder (MDD) patients, normal morning but elevated evening plasma cortisol levels were found in patients with GAD compared to those with MDD. In another study, GAD patients who had received 48 cognitive therapy sessions had a significant decrease in afternoon cortisol levels, but not in GAD symptoms after 24 weeks compared to untreated controls in whom the levels remained the same (Tafet *et al.* 2005).

4.3.3 Noradrenergic (NE) system

Although the exact pathophysiological role of the NE system in GAD is unclear, it has been well established that the NE plays a key role in models of acute and chronic stress as well as in the constructs of sensitization and fear conditioning.

Platelet monoamine oxidase activity is increased in patients with GAD and a hyporesponsive and prolonged autonomic response has been demonstrated in skin conductance tests in GAD. Studies measuring plasma levels of NE and free 3-methoxy-4 hydroxyphenylethylene glycol or catechol-*O*-methyl transferase of dopamine β-hydroxylase are equivocal as some have indicated an increase in NE activity and others have found no difference between GAD subjects and normal controls. Studies examining the inhibitory α_2-adrenoreceptor have also been inconsistent. In animal studies, inhibition of these receptors presynaptically led to increased NE activity but this was not found in GAD subjects who have been treated with α_2-adrenoreceptor antagonists (Jetty *et al.* 2001).

In most of the studies examining NE function in GAD, older diagnostic criteria were used which limits the generalizability of the findings. This, coupled with inconsistent evidence of the role of the NE system in GAD, indicates further research is necessary to address the role of this system in GAD.

4.3.4 Serotonin (5-HT)

Serotonin (5-HT) function has long been presumed to play a role in the pathogenesis of GAD based upon the efficacy of serotonergic agents (e.g., serotonin re-uptake inhibitors (SSRIs)) for this condition. 'Knock-out mice' bred without $5-HT_{1A}$ receptors show decreased exploratory behaviour and increased fear of aversive stimuli, furthermore studies of $5-HT_{1A}$ receptor agonists have demonstrated their effectiveness in treating GAD.

In clinical studies, evidence such as reduced serotonin levels in the cerebrospinal fluid, decreased platelet paroxetine binding and higher levels of both urinary lysosomal enzyme N-acetyl-β-glucosaminidase and 5-hydroxyindoleacetic acid (a 5-HT metabolite) support the potential role of serotonin in GAD. Recent investigations have focused on the involvement of particular 5-HT receptor subtypes in GAD and anxiety. The roles of $5-HT_1$, $5-HT_{2A}$, and $5-HT_{2C}$ receptors in pathologic anxiety have been suggested in part through studies demonstrating the efficacy of agents affecting them including buspirone ($5-HT_1$ partial agonist) and nefazodone ($5-HT_2$ blocker). However, the nature of serotonergic abnormalities relevant to anxiety remains uncertain with evidence suggesting both hyperactive or hypoactive function (Jetty *et al.* 2001).

4.3.5 Benzodiazepine receptors

Clinical studies support the role of benzodiazepine receptor dysfunction in anxiogenesis and indicate that GAD may be associated with an abnormal decrease in peripheral lymphocyte benzodiazepine receptors (PBR). This finding has also been seen in OCD but not in panic disorder, suggesting that changes in lymphocyte PBR may distinguish between different types of anxiety states. Other relevant findings of a concurrent decrease in relative mRNA encoding PBR indicate that the rate of synthesis of these receptors may also be decreased when illness is active, and reversed with successful treatment.

4.3.6 Sodium lactate and carbon dioxide

Sodium lactate and carbon dioxide challenge studies have provided interesting information concerning the differentiation of PD and GAD. Overall, patients with GAD and PD responded differently from each other to these challenges, though both tend to be more responsive than normal controls For example, patients with GAD had lower rates of panic attacks post-lactate infusion when compared to PD patients. PD patients showed a greater subjective response to inhaling carbon dioxide than GAD patients, but the response of both groups was greater than that of normal controls. These studies may suggest that GAD and PD are distinct disorders which share a common sensitivity to physiological stressors (Jetty et al. 2001).

4.4 Genetics and heritability

The bulk of studies examining genetics and heritability in anxiety disorders have tended to focus on PD, obsessive compulsive disorder, and to some extent social phobia. Few studies have focused on GAD and available literature shows discordant opinions regarding the influence of genetics on GAD. Much of the current literature has examined GAD and MDD in an effort to distinguish them as separate disorders.

4.4.1 Family studies

Family studies have indicated that GAD is transmitted familially. One study found that 19.5% of first-degree relatives of GAD (DSM-III) probands had developed the disorder compared with only 3.5% of relatives of control subjects' with a corresponding relative risk of 5.6 (large compared to other anxiety disorders). In another study, GAD was diagnosed in 22% of first-degree relatives of 33 probands with anxiety disorders (where 13 of these probands had GAD) indicating no evidence of inheritance (Jetty et al. 2001). Twin and adoption studies have also been equivocal. In the large Virginia twin study and Swedish twin registry of GAD and depression (Kendler et al. 1992; Roy et al. 1995), genetic factors appeared to account for both GAD and MDD. However, an index monozygote with one of the disorders was found to be just as likely to have a twin with either disorder. In a follow-up study it was found that GAD had about a 30% heritability rate. This sample was the largest to date with 2,352 female twin subjects. Findings were subject to criticism, however, because the authors loosened diagnostic criteria to obtain a larger sample size; nevertheless the results were suggestive of an identical genetic liability between MDD and GAD and that the specific disorder developed is determined entirely by environmental factors (Jetty et al. 2001).

In contrast, a family study of co-transmission of alcoholism, depression, and anxiety disorders found that more than half the variance in liability for GAD and depression may be accounted for by extra-familial influences and may not be caused by a shared environment (Merikangas et al. 1994). Furthermore, another family study found that lifetime co-occurrence of GAD and PD could not be explained by family environmental influences (Scherrer et al. 2000). Although far from definitive, the current evidence suggests that MDD and

GAD may share an overlapping genotype; however, the expression of these disorders seems largely dependent upon environmental factors.

4.4.2 Molecular genetic studies

To date, there have been no genome studies specific to GAD. An association between several single nucleotide polymorphisms (SNP) has been found in a *GAD1* gene encoding glutamic acid decarboxylase enzymes, which are responsible for synthesizing gamma-aminobutyric acid (GABA) into glutamate (Gelernter and Stein 2008). The 5-HT transporter gene (located on chromosome 17q) has demonstrated significantly higher proportions of the *Stin2.12* allele in GAD versus normal controls. Similar results have been found in OCD and MDD (Ohara *et al.* 1999).

4.5 Conclusion

Studies examining the neurobiology of GAD remain inconclusive although data are accruing that may be informative. There is some suggestion of insula activation in GAD which interestingly maps well onto the concept of intolerance of uncertainty that is discussed in the cognitive behavioural literature (Chapter 6). The pharmacological treatment literature suggests that the NE, serotonergic, and GABAergic systems may be involved in GAD, although abnormalities in the direct measures or correlates of these neurotransmitters are only mildly supportive of this assertion. Further neuroimaging studies of adults with GAD are necessary to help better understand the CNS structures involved in the genesis and maintenance of GAD. Genetic studies using techniques such as candidate gene strategies and studies of complex trait genetics will likely yield increased understanding of the neurobiological underpinnings of GAD.

References

Britton JC, Rauch SL. (2008). Neuroanatomy and neuroimaging of anxiety disorders, in: Antony MM, Stein MB (Eds). *Oxford Handbook of Anxiety and Related Disorders.* Oxford University Press, Oxford.

Gelernter J, Stein MB. (2008). Heritability and genetics of anxiety disorders, in: Antony MM, Stein MB (Eds). *Oxford Handbook of Anxiety and Related Disorders.* Oxford University Press, Oxford.

Jetty PV, Charnet DS, Goddard AW. (2001). Neurobiology of generalized anxiety disorder. *Psych Clin N Am,* **24**, 71–97.

Kendler KS, Neale MC, Kessler RC, Heath AC, Eaves LJ. (1992). Major depression and generalized anxiety disorder: Same genes (partly) different environments? *Arch Gen Psych,* **49**, 716–22.

McClure EB, Monk CS, Nelson EE et al. (2007). Abnormal alteration modulation of fear circuit function in pediatric generalized anxiety disorder. *Arch Gen Psychiatry*, **64**, 97–106.

Merikangas KR, Risch NJ, Weissman MM. (1994). Comorbidity and co-transmission of alcoholism, anxiety and depression. *Psychol Med*, **24**, 69–80.

Monk CS, Nelson EE, McClure EB et al. (2006). Ventrolateral prefrontal cortex activation and attentional bias in response to angry faces in adolescents with generalized anxiety disorder. *Am J Psych*, **163**, 1091–7.

Ohara K, Suzuki Y, Ochiai M, Tsukamoto T, Tani K, Ohara K. (1999). A variable-number-tandem-repeat of the serotonin transporter gene and anxiety disorders. *Prog Neuropsychopharmacol Biol Psychiatry* **23**, 55–65.

Paulesu E, Sambugaro E, Torti T et al. (2010). Neural correlates of worry in generalized anxiety disorder and in normal controls: a functional MRI study. *Psychol Med*, **40**, 117–24.

Roy MA, Neale MC, Pedersen NL, Mathe AA, Kendler KS. (1995). A twin study of generalized anxiety disorder and major depression. *Psychol Med*, **25**, 1037–49.

Scherrer JF, True WR, Xianb H et al. (2000). Evidence for genetic influences common and specific to symptoms of generalized anxiety and panic. *J Affect Disord*, **57**, 25–35.

Simmons A, Matthews SC, Paulus MP, Stein MB. (2008). Intolerance of uncertainty correlates with insula activation during affective ambiguity. *Neurosci Lett*, **430**, 92–7.

Tafet GE, Feder DJ, Abulafia DP, Roffman SS. (2005). Regulation of hypothalamic-pituitary-adrenal activity in response to cognitive therapy in patients with generalized anxiety disorder. *Cognitive, Affective, Behavioral Neurosci*, **5**, 37–40.

Tafet GE, Toister-Achituv M, Shinitzky M. (2001). Enhancement of serotonin uptake by cortisol: A possible link between stress and depression. *Cognitive, Affective Behavioral Neurosci*, **1**, 96–104.

Thomas KM, Drevets WC, Dahl RE et al. (2001). Amygdala response to fearful faces in anxious and depressed children. *Arch Gen Psych*, **58**, 1057–63.

Willour VL, Yao SY, Samuels J et al. (2004). Replication study supports evidence for linkage to 9p24 in obsessive-compulsive disorder. *Am J Hum Genet*, **75**, 508–13.

Chapter 5

Pharmacotherapy

Michael Van Ameringen and Mark H. Pollack

> **Key points**
>
> - A broad range of agents have been found to be efficacious in the treatment of generalized anxiety disorder (GAD).
> - Selective serotonin re-uptake inhibitors, serotonin noradrenaline re-uptake inhibitors, pregabalin, and the benzodiazepines are typical first-line pharmacological treatments.
> - First-line agents have been shown to be effective in the long-term and to prevent relapse.
> - There are few evidence-based strategies for treatment of refractory GAD, but augmentation with atypical antipsychotics, benzodiazepines, pregabalin, or cognitive-behavioural therapy may be helpful.

5.1 Introduction

The evaluation of pharmacological treatments for generalized anxiety disorder (GAD) has spanned a broad range of drug classes. Benzodiazepines have long been the mainstay of the treatment of GAD; however, selective serotonin re-uptake inhibitors (SSRIs) and serotonin-noradrenaline re-uptake inhibitors (SNRIs) have emerged as the gold standard treatments over the last decade. Anticonvulsants have been increasingly used for the treatment of GAD and other anxiety disorders as well. Other agents including azapirones, beta-blockers, antihistamines have also been evaluated in GAD. The current evidence for the efficacy of pharmacotherapy across a variety of drug classes in GAD will be reviewed in this chapter.

5.2 Pharmacotherapy of GAD by drug class

A summary of randomized controlled trials (RCT) of pharmacotherapy in GAD is provided in Table 5.1 (Van Ameringen *et al.* in press; Mathew and Hoffman 2009).

Table 5.1 Randomized controlled trials of pharmacotherapy in GAD

Drug, class and study		N	Weeks	Design	Efficacy
			Acute trials		
Selective serotonin re-uptake inhibitors (SSRIs)					
Escitalopram	Davidson et al. (2004)	307	8	ESC(10–20mg/day) vs. PBO	ESC > PBO
	Goodman et al. (2005)	856	8	ESC (10–20 mg/day) vs. PBO	ESC > PBO
	Baldwin et al (2006)	681	12	ESC (5, 10, 20 mg/day) vs. PAR (20 mg/day) vs. PBO	ESC (10, 20 mg/d) > PAR (20 mg/d) = ESC (5 mg/day) > PBO
Paroxetine	Rocca et al. (1997)	81	8	PAR (20 mg/day) vs. IMP (50–100 mg/day) vs. DIA (3–6 mg/day)	PAR = IMP = DIA
	Hewitt et al. (2001)	364	8	PAR (20–50 mg/day) vs. PBO	PAR = PBO
	Pollack et al. (2001)	324	8	PAR (20–50 mg/day) vs. PBO	PAR >PBO
	Rickels et al. (2003)	566	8	PAR (20, 40 mg/day) vs. PBO	PAR > PBO
Sertraline	Morris et al. (2003)	188	12	SER (50–150 mg/day) vs. PBO	SER > PBO
	Sjodin et al. (2003)	188	12	SER (50–150 mg/day) vs. PBO	SER > PBO *Primary outcome was quality of life assessment*
	Allgulander et al. (2004)	330	12	SER (50–150 mg/day) vs. PBO	SER > PBO
	Ball et al. (2005)	55	8	SER (25–100 mg/day) vs. PAR (10–40 mg/day) vs. PBO	SER = PAR > PBO

	Steiner et al. (2005)	370	12	SER (50–150 mg/day) vs. PBO	SER > PBO
	Brawman-Mintzer et al. (2006)	326	10	SER (50–200 mg/day) vs. PBO	SER > PBO

Serotonin noradrenaline re-uptake inhibitors (SNRIs)

Venlafaxine ER	Davidson et al. (1999)	365	8	VEN (75, 150 mg/day) vs. BUS (30 mg/day) vs. PBO	VEN > PBO and BUS > PBO on some measures
	Rickels et al. (2000)	377	8	VEN (75, 150, 225 mg/day) vs. PBO	VEN (225 mg/day) > PBO (4 of 4 primary outcome) VEN (150 mg/day) > PBO (1 of 4 primary outcome)
	Nimatoudis et al. (2004)	46	8	VEN (75, 150 mg/day) vs. PBO	VEN > PBO
	Kim et al. (2006)	60	8	VEN (37.5–225 mg/day) vs. PAR (10–40 mg/day)	VEN = PAR
Duloxetine	Allgulander et al. (2007) (3 studies -pooled analysis)	1163	9–10	DUL (60–120 mg/day) vs. PBO DUL (60, 120 mg/day) vs PBO	DUL > PBO DUL > PBO
	Allgulander et al. (2008) (2 studies-pooled analysis)	984	10	DUL (20–120 mg/day) vs. PBO VEN (75–225 mg/day) vs. PBO	DUL = VEN > PBO

Tricyclic antidepressants (TCA)

Imipramine	Hoehn-Saric et al. (1988)	52	6	IMP (25–300 mg/day) vs. ALP (1.5–6 mg/day)	IMP = ALP
	Rickels et al. (1993)	230	8	IMP (25–200 mg/day) vs. TRA (50–400 mg/day) vs. DIA (5–40 mg/day) vs. PBO	IMP = TRA = DIA >PBO

Table 5.1 (Contd.)

Drug, class and study		Acute trials		
	N	Weeks	Design	Efficacy
TCAs *continued*				
Opipramol				
Moller et al. (2001) (ICD-10 criteria)	310	4	OPI (200 mg/day) vs. ALP (2 mg/day) vs. PBO	OPI = ALP > PBO
Other antidepressants				
Agomelatine				
Stein et al. (2007)	121	12	AGO (20–50 mg/day) vs. PBO	AGO > PBO
Bupropion XL				
Bystritsky et al. (2008)	32	12	BUP (300 mg/day) vs. ESC (20 mg/day) vs. PBO	BUP > ESC
Anticonvulsants				
Pregabalin				
Feltner et al. (2003)	271	4	PRE (150 mg/day) vs. PRE (600 mg/day) vs. LOR (6 mg/day) vs. PBO	PRE (600 mg/day) > PBO LOR > PBO
Pande et al. (2003)	276	6	PRE (150, 600 mg/day) vs. LOR (6 mg/day) vs. PBO	PRE (600 mg/day) = LOR > PBO
Pohl et al. (2005)	341	6	PRE (200, 400, 450 mg/day) vs. PBO	PRE > PBO
Rickels et al. (2005)	454	4	PRE (300, 450, 600 mg/day) vs. ALP (4.5 mg/day) vs. PBO	PRE = ALP > PBO
Montgomery et al. (2006)	421	6	PRE (400, 600 mg/day) vs. VEN (75 mg/day) vs. PBO	PRE = VEN > PBO
Kasper et al. (2009)	374	8	PRE (300–600 mg/day) vs. VEN (75–225 mg/day) vs. PBO	PRE > VEN = PBO

Tiagabine	Pollack et al. (2005)	272	8	TIA (mean 10.5 mg/day) vs. PBO	TIA = PBO
	Pollack et al. (2008) (pooled analysis)	1790	10	TIA (4, 8, 12 mg/day) vs. PBO TIA (4–16 mg/day) vs. PBO TIA (4–16 mg/day) vs. PBO	TIA = PBO TIA = PBO TIA = PBO
Antipsychotics					
Trifluorperazine	Mendels et al. (1986)	415	4	TRI (2–6 mg/day) vs. PBO	TRI > PBO
Quetiapine	Brawman-Mintzer et al. (2006)	38	6	QUE (25–300 mg/day) vs. PBO	QUE = PBO
	Chouinard et al. (2007)	873	8	QUE (50, 150 mg/day) vs. PAR (20 mg/day) vs. PBO	QUE (50,150 mg/day) > PBO PAR > PBO
	Joyce et al. (2008)	951	8	QUE (50, 150, 300 mg/day) vs. PBO	QUE (50,150 mg/day) > PBO QUE (300 mg/day) = PBO
	Merideth et al. (2008)	854	10	QUE (150, 300 mg/day) vs (ESC 10 mg/day) vs. PBO	QUE (150, 300 mg/day) > PBO ESC > PBO
Azapirones					
Buspirone	Cohn et al. (1989)	367	4	BUS (10–60 mg/day) vs. DIA (10–60 mg/day) vs. PBO	BUS = DIA > PBO
	Ansseau et al. (1990)	26	6	BUS (15 mg/day) vs. OXA (45 mg/day)	OXA > BUS
	Enkelmann (1991)	94	6	BUS (15–40 mg/day) vs. ALP (1.5–4 mg/day) vs. PBO	ALP > BUS > PBO

Table 5.1 (Contd.)

Drug, class and study	Acute trials			
	N	Weeks	Design	Efficacy
Tollefson et al. (1992) (recovering alcoholics)	51	24	BUS (30–60 mg/day) vs. PBO	BUS > PBO
Sramrek et al. (1996)	162	6	BUS (15–45 mg/day) vs. PBO	BUS > PBO
Sramek et al. (1997)	119	8	BUS (15mg BID) vs. BUS (10mg TID) vs. PBO	BUS > PBO BUS BID = BUS TID
Laakmann et al. (1998)	125	10	BUS (15 mg/day) vs. LOR (3 mg/day) vs. PBO	BUS = LOR > PBO
Majercsik et al. (2003)	52	6	BUS (30 mg/day) vs. PBO	BUS > PBO
Benzodiazepines[†]				
Fontaine et al. (1983)	48	4	BRO (18 mg/day) vs. DIA (15 mg/day) vs. PBO	BRO > DIA > PBO
Fontaine et al. (1986)	60	4	BRO (12,18 mg/day) vs. LOR (4, 6 mg/day) vs. PBO	BRO = LOR > PBO
Rickels et al. (1998)	62	4	CLO (15–30 mg/day) vs. LOR (2–4 mg/day)	CLO = LOR

Antihistamines				
Hydroxyzine	Darcis et al. (1995)	100	4	HYD (50 mg/day) vs. PBO	HYD > PBO
	Lader and Scotto (1998)	214	4	HYD (50 mg/day) vs. BUS (20 mg/day) vs. PBO	HYD > BUS = PBO
	Llorca et al. (2002)	334	12	HYD (50 mg/day) vs. BRO (6 mg/day) vs. PBO	HYD = BRO > PBO
Beta blockers					
Atenolol	Rickels et al. (1986)	63	3	ATN (100 mg/day) vs. PBO	ATN = PBO
Propranolol	Meibach et al. (1987)	212	3	PRO (80, 160, 320 mg/day) vs. CHL (30, 45, 75 mg/day) vs. PBO	PRO = CHL = PBO

Abbreviations (alphabetical): ABE = abecarnil; AGO = agomelatine; ALP = alprazolam; ATN = atenolol; BRO = bromazepam; BUP = bupropion XL; BUS = buspirone; CHL = chlordiazepoxide; CLO = clorazepate; DIA = diazepam; DUL = duloxetine; ESC = escitalopram; HYD = hyroxyzine; IMP = imipramine; LES = lesopitron; LOR = lorazepam; OPI = opipramol; OXA = oxazepam; PAR = paroxetine; PBO = placebo; PRO = propranolol; PRE = pregabalin; QUE = quetiapine; SER = sertraline; TIA = tiagabine; TRA = trazodone; TRI = trifluoperazine; VEN = venlafaxine ER

† The examination of benzodiazepines in DSM-III, III-R and IV GAD has mainly been through comparisons with other medications: paroxetine (one study), imipramine (three studies), opipramol (one study), pregabalin (three studies), buspirone (four studies), hydroxyzine (one study) and propranolol (one study). These studies are outlined in their respective sections of Table 5.1. For a more comprehensive review please see Van Ameringen et al. (in press).

5.2.1 **Benzodiazepines**

Benzodiazepines continue to be the most commonly prescribed anxiolytic medications and have a long history of use in the treatment of GAD. Benzodiazepines enhance the effects of the inhibitory neurotransmitter gamma-aminobutyric acid (GABA), through their binding to specific receptors on the GABA receptor complex, causing an overall decrease in psychological and physiological arousal. Chlordiazepoxide, diazepam, clorazepate, lorazepam, and oxazepam have all been shown to be more efficacious than placebo for the treatment of non-specific anxiety symptoms (Greenblatt and Shader 1974). More specific research regarding the treatment of GAD includes positive placebo RCT's of clorazepate, lorazepam, bromazepam, and diazepam. These positive results were obtained in patient populations defined by the DSM-III GAD criteria but are still likely relevant for patients defined by current diagnostic criteria.

Comparator trials using the anticonvulsant agent pregabalin were the first RCTs of benzodiazepines using DSM-IV criteria in GAD. Results of these RCTs indicated that alprazolam and lorazepam were superior to placebo.

Despite their demonstrated efficacy, rapid onset of effect, low cost given their generic status, and generally favourable side-effect profile in GAD, benzodiazepine administration may be associated with a number of disadvantages. The half-life of some benzodiazepines (e.g. alprazolam, lorazepam) is relatively short, requiring two to four times per day dosing and sometimes resulting in interdose rebound anxiety. Moreover, some data suggest that when compared to antidepressants, benzodiazepines may be associated with high rates of relapse following treatment discontinuation. Other drawbacks to these agents include the potential for rebound anxiety and other withdrawal symptomatology associated with discontinuation, as well as their potential for abuse in patients with a predisposition towards substance abuse. Other potential side effects of benzodiazepines include attentional, psychomotor, cognitive, and memory effects. Benzodiazepines lack the broad spectrum efficacy of antidepressants in the treatment of common co-morbid conditions such as depression and thus may not be appropriate monotherapy for the majority of anxious patients who have significant concurrent depression.

5.2.2 **Antidepressants**

5.2.2.1 *Tricyclic antidepressants (TCAs)*

TCAs work by inhibiting the re-uptake of neurotransmitters including norepinephrine and serotonin. The prototypic TCA, imipramine, has established efficacy for the treatment of GAD in an RCT. Other TCAs are likely effective as well although there is little systematic data addressing this issue. Like all antidepressants, onset of therapeutic effects is not typically observed for at least 2 to 3 weeks and some-times longer.

Opipramol, a drug widely prescribed in Germany (but not available in North America or UK), is a tricyclic compound which is an effective D2, 5HT2, and H1 receptor blocker and has no re-uptake-inhibiting properties. Results from a GAD study comparing opipramol to alpra-zolam and placebo indicated that both active agents were superior to placebo and equal in efficacy to each other.

However, the use of the TCAs is associated with a significant side-effect burden including sedation, weight gain, orthostasis, and antimuscarinic effects attributable to blockade at H1 histamine, α1-adrenoceptors, and muscarinic receptors. In addition, they have adverse effects on cardiac conduction and are potentially lethal in overdose. Thus although of equivalent efficacy to newer antidepres-sants (SSRIs and SNRIs) and lacking the abuse and dependence potential associated with the benzodiazepines, they have largely been supplanted as first-line agents for GAD (and other disorders) by the SSRIs and SNRIs.

5.2.2.2 *Selective serotonin re-uptake inhibitors*

The primary mechanism of action of the SSRIs is through blockade of the re-uptake of serotonin. Based on the strong efficacy of these agents found in RCTs, their broad spectrum of action on co-morbid conditions, as well as their safety and tolerability profiles, SSRIs are considered first-line agents in the treatment of GAD.

Escitalopram has been shown to be effective in short-term trials (up to 12 weeks), long-term trials (up to 76 weeks), and relapse prevention studies.

The efficacy of paroxetine in the treatment of GAD has been demonstrated in short-term trials, in comparator trials with escitalo-pram, imipramine, diazepam, venlafaxine, and sertraline, and relapse prevention studies.

Treatment with sertraline in GAD has been examined in five short-term RCTs, including one comparator study (to paroxetine) all of which have been positive. One of these studies evaluated efficacy according to gender and found no difference.

5.2.2.3 *Serotonin-noradrenaline re-uptake inhibitors*

The primary mechanism of action of SNRIs is the selective, dose-dependent blockade of serotonin and noradrenaline re-uptake. The novel SNRI, venlafaxine modified release has demonstrated efficacy for the treatment of GAD as evidenced by results from several RCTs. There have been four short-term placebo-controlled RCTs, of venlafaxine in GAD. Two of these studies had active comparators, one with buspirone and the other with pregabalin. All of these stud-ies found venlafaxine significantly better than placebo and at least equally effective to the comparator drug. In addition, there is one comparator study which found equal efficacy with paroxetine. The efficacy of venlafaxine has also been evaluated in long-term trials (up to 28 weeks) and in childhood GAD. Duloxetine is another dual re-uptake inhibitor of both serotonin and norepinephrine. It has been studied in three short-term placebo-controlled RCT studies, one of which had an active comparator (venlafaxine). In a pooled analysis of the three short-term studies (over 1,100 patients), duloxetine was found to have a significant reduction of anxiety symptoms on the primary outcome measure (HAMA), significantly higher response rates and a greater degree of improvement in functional impairment over placebo (Allgulander *et al.* 2007).

5.2.3 Other antidepressants

5.2.3.1 *Agomelatine*

Agomelatine has a novel mechanism of action, primarily affecting the hormone melatonin which is involved in the maintenance of circadian rhythms. Agomelatine acts as a MT1 and MT2 agonist and also as a 5HT2C antagonist. In the only randomized, double-blind, placebo-controlled study to date, it was found that at study end point agome-latine patients had significantly higher response (≥50% HAMA reduc-tion) and remission rates (HAMA ≤7) than for placebo controls. Agomelatine-treated patients did not differ significantly from placebo controls in the incidence of treatment-related adverse events or discontinuation symptoms. Agomelatine displayed a favourable toler-ability profile when compared to traditional antidepressants and may prove to be a useful treatment option for GAD.

5.2.3.2 *Bupropion*

Bupropion is an antidepressant which acts as a norephinephrine and dopamine re-uptake inhibitor. This agent belongs to the class of aminoketones and is similar in structure to phenethylamines. In a small double-blind, controlled comparison study of outpatients with GAD, bupropion m/r showed comparable efficacy to escitalopram. These results suggest the potential utility of bupropion in the treat-ment of GAD, though the findings need to be confirmed in large placebo-controlled studies.

5.2.4 Antipsychotics

First-generation antipsychotic medications have been used for many years for the treatment of anxiety. Trifluoroperazine showed positive data in one RCT (Mendels *et al.* 1986) and obtained FDA approval for short-term treatment of non-psychotic anxiety. However, the use of antipsychotics in practice has been constrained by concerns about their potential to cause extra-pyramidal symptoms (EPS) and tardive dyskinesia (TD) (Seeman 2002).

The second generation or so-called atypical antipsychotics are less likely to cause EPS or TD than first-generation agents and have a variety of effects on serotonin receptors believed relevant to anxiolysis which has encouraged exploration of their use for the treatment of GAD. The atypicals have been found to be effective in the treatment of bipolar disorder and refractory depression suggesting potential utility for the treatment of individuals with co-morbid anxiety and mood disorders, particularly those refractory to standard interventions.

Studies of quetiapine in acute monotherapy in non-refractory GAD have been primarily positive (one study was negative). Three of the studies were fixed dose and two of these studies had active comparators, one with paroxetine, one with escitalopram, and both comparators were also superior to placebo.

The usual dose range for atypicals in the treatment of GAD is typically lower than doses employed in psychotic disorders (e.g. 2.5 to 10 mg/day olanzapine; 0.5 to 3 mg/day risperidone; 2 to 15 mg/day aripiprazole; 50 to 300 mg/day quetiapine). The onset of therapeutic effect is often within a week or two after treatment initiation.

Based on the emerging evidence regarding the efficacy of antipsychotics in the treatment of GAD, these agents appear promising especially for those patients who are resistant to or unable to tolerate standard GAD treatments. However, given the association of second-generation antipsychotics with adverse effects including weight gain, hyperglycaemia, diabetes, hyperlipidaemia, and other manifestations of metabolic syndrome, clinicians using these agents should familiarize themselves with the recommendations for baseline and ongoing monitoring of treated patients for these adverse effects (Barrett 2004).

5.2.5 Anticonvulsants

Abnormalities in GABA (inhibitory) systems and glutamatergic (excitatory) systems have been associated with various anxiety disorders. A dysfunction in GABA-A receptor binding is also thought to play a role in anxiety disorders, stemming from the observation of diminished response to exogenous benzodiazepines in individuals with anxiety. Various anticonvulsant agents are thought to modulate GABAergic and glutamatergic systems, and therefore treating anxious patients with such agents may restore the homeostasis between these two neurotransmitters and decrease neuronal overexcitability, particularly in areas relevant for genesis of anxiety such as the amygdala.

Pregabalin is a structural analogue to GABA, although it is not active at GABA receptors, nor does it acutely alter GABA uptake or degradation. It has a novel mechanism of action, binding to the delta subunit of voltage-dependent calcium channels in CNS and acting as a presynaptic modulator of several excitatory neurotransmitters.

Pregabalin was evaluated in five short-term acute studies in GAD. All of these studies compared two or three dose levels of pregabalin to placebo. In four of the five trials an active comparator was used (i.e. lorazepam, alprazolam, and venlafaxine). All of the studies demonstrated pregabalin to be significantly superior to placebo and equally effective to the comparator agent including a similar speed of therapeutic onset to the benzodiazepine comparator. Common side effects included somnolence and dizziness. This finding was confirmed by Lydiard et al. (2010) in a pooled analysis. Pregabalin is currently indicated for the treatment of GAD in Europe, though not in the USA or Canada. Further study of its ability to treat common co-morbid conditions, including depressive symptoms and other anxiety disorders, and further comparator trials would facilitate a fuller assessment of its relative role in the GAD pharmacopoeia.

Tiagabine is a selective GABA re-uptake inhibitor (SGRI). It increases the synaptic GABA availability by selective inhibition of the GAT-1 GABA transporter, the most abundant GABA transporter. It is indicated as an add-on treatment of partial seizures. Although one large 8-week double-blind, placebo-controlled trial examining tiagabine monotherapy in GAD suggested potential efficacy for this agent, a subsequent combined analysis of three further RCTs (one fixed dose and two flexible dose), showed no significant effect for the active agent, and did not support its consideration as an effective anxiolytic.

5.2.6 Other medications

5.2.6.1 *Azapirones*

Buspirone, an azapirone derivative, is a partial 5-HT1A receptor agonist that has been approved in the USA by the Food and Drug Administration for the treatment of generalized anxiety since 1986. It has demonstrated efficacy in a number of clinical trials and has a generally favourable side-effect profile. The benefits of buspirone include a low potential for abuse or dependence; negligible toxicity in overdose; an absence of respiratory depressant properties; no serious drug interaction effects; limited sedation; a lack of cognitive, memory or psychomotor adverse effects; and no antimuscarinic or cardiotoxic effects. Its use may be associated with dizziness or gastrointestinal distress (Napoliello and Domantay 1991). Despite its tolerability and demonstrable efficacy in clinical trials, it has been considered inconsistently effective in clinical practice, limiting its widespread use as anti-anxiety monotherapy, although it may have some application as an augmentation agent for first-line anxiolytics.

5.2.6.2 *Beta-blockers*

Beta-blockers (e.g. propranolol and atenolol) block the action of catecholamines on both β1- and β2-adrenergic receptors, potentially producing anxiolytic effects. Although the limited systematic data available (two negative studies) do not support their routine use as primary anxiolytics, beta-blockers are sometimes used as an augmentation strategy to treat persistent symptoms of autonomic arousal (e.g. tachycardia, tremor) for patients on standard anti-anxiety treatments.

5.2.6.3 *Antihistamines*

Hydroxyzine is an H1-receptor antagonist, as well as a weak 5HT2 receptor antagonist, and has been shown to possess some anxiolytic properties. To date, there are only a handful of RCTs examining the effectiveness of hydroxyzine in GAD. Although the results of RCTs demonstrate the efficacy of hydroxyzine in GAD, it is not typically used as a first- or second-line agent due to its significant sedative properties and the lack of demonstrated efficacy in common co-morbid conditions found with GAD. It is typically used as an augmentation or alternative strategy for patients refractory to or intolerant of standard interventions.

5.3 Safety and adverse events

5.3.1 Antidepressants
5.3.1.1 *SSRIs and SNRIs*

SSRIs and SNRIs are generally better tolerated than the older classes of antidepressants but are still associated with treatment emergent adverse effects. Overstimulation characterized by increased anxiety symptoms, jitteriness, motor restlessness, insomnia, and headaches can commonly occur at the beginning of treatment, but may be prevented or reduced by starting at a low dose and using a slow upward dose titration. Sleep disturbances and gastrointestinal side effects are common side effects seen with SSRIs and SNRIs. Sweating and headaches are also common early in treatment; sexual dysfunction and weight gain may occur with treatment over time. There is also potential for an emergent withdrawal syndrome to occur during antidepressant discontinuation, which may be ameliorated with a slow and gradual taper regimen. In addition to a side-effect profile comparable to the SSRIs, the SNRI venlafaxine m/r may be associated with increased blood pressure particularly at higher doses, and duloxetine may be associated with urinary retention.

5.3.1.2 *Monoamine oxidase inhibitors*

Monoamine oxidase inhibitors (MAOIs) are typically reserved for patients remaining symptomatic despite other interventions. This is due to their more adverse side-effect profile, the critical dietary, and concomitant drug restrictions and because of the potential for emergent hypertensive crises and serotonin syndrome. MAOIs are usually given in the morning and at mid-day to reduce associated insomnia.

5.3.1.3 *Tricyclic antidepressants*

As with the SSRIs and SNRIs, there is the risk of overstimulation. Most TCAs have antimuscarinic properties which can lead to bothersome adverse events such as dry mouth, blurred vision, postural hypotension, tachycardia, sedation, sexual dysfunction, and impaired psychomotor functioning. Weight gain can also occur with prolonged use. A discontinuation syndrome has been reported with abrupt cessation of TCAs. TCAs can be associated with cardiac rhythm disturbances and may be lethal in overdose, a significant issue for patients at risk for suicidality.

5.3.2 **Benzodiazepines**

Benzodiazepines have a generally favourable side-effect profile though they may be associated with sedation, dizziness, cognitive and memory impairment, as well as psychomotor impairment. After 3 or 4 weeks of regular use, physiologic dependence may develop, necessitating the need for gradual taper to avoid significant withdrawal reactions when discontinuation is attempted. Patients with a predisposition to alcohol, benzodiazepine, or psychoactive substance abuse or dependence are at risk to abuse benzodiazepines and should be treated with alternatives when possible. Long-term use of benzodiazepines does not usually lead to tolerance to the anxiolytic effects.

5.3.3 **5HT1a agonists**

Buspirone is a generally well-tolerated non-benzodiazepine anxiolytic. Side effects are usually minimal but can include headache dizziness, light-headedness, restlessness, fatigue, nervousness, nausea, and sweating.

5.3.4 **Antihistamines**

Hydroxyzine is not generally used as a first-line agent, due to its inconsistent efficacy and side-effect profile which includes excessive sedation and weight gain. Antimuscarinic effects can occur at high doses, leading to dry mouth, blurred vision, confusion, and even delirium.

5.3.5 **Antipsychotics**

Conventional antipsychotics are now infrequently used for the treatment of anxiety disorders due to concerns about extra-pyramidal effects and TD. Although the atypical antipsychotics are generally better tolerated than the newer agents with a lower risk of treatment emergent movement disorders, they may be associated with an array of significant side effects which require careful monitoring including weight gain, changes in glucose and lipid levels, diabetes, and elevated prolactin, as well as sedation, orthostatic hypotension, extra-pyramidal effects, and sexual dysfunction.

Atypical antipsychotics are currently not used as first-line agents for the treatment for GAD, but are reserved for treatment resistant cases and as an 'add-on' treatment.

5.3.6 Anticonvulsants

Pregablin is the only anticonvulsant that has supportive evidence for use in GAD. Pregabalin can be associated with dizziness, somnolence, peripheral oedema, and dry mouth.

5.4 Comparative efficacy

Head to head studies of anxyolytic agents have been equal in efficacy; however, these studies are generally not designed with a significant sample size to show a difference between the index drug and the active comparator. Another way to evaluate comparative efficacy is through a statistical technique, known as the meta-analysis. In a recent meta-analysis of 21 double-blind placebo-controlled trials of medications treating DSM-III-R, DSM-IV, or ICD-10 GAD, the efficacy of a variety of agents was compared, using the change in HAM-A score from baseline to end point as the main efficacy measure. Based on the results of these meta-analyses (Table 5.2), pregabalin was found to have the greatest effect size (see footnote*); however, in addition to pregabalin, the SSRIs and SNRIs were recommended to be first-line treatment due to their reasonable effect size, broad spectrum of efficacy across common co-morbid conditions, and good tolerability.

5.5 Long-term GAD treatment

As GAD tends to be a chronic and recurrent condition, demonstration of the long-term benefit of pharmacotherapy is critical. This has been evaluated in both long-term controlled studies and relapse prevention studies.

5.6 Long-term studies

Venlafaxine, escitalopram, paroxetine, buspirone, clorazepate, and diazepam have all been examined in long-term studies (Table 5.3). There have been three studies evaluating the long-term efficacy of

---

* Effect size (ES) is a measure of the magnitude of treatment effect across several studies as compared to a control treatment. It is statistical method frequently used in meta-analyses which summarizes several studies into a single estimate after a standard measure of effect has been calculated for each study. The ES is roughly the difference between the mean values of the two groups, divided by the standard deviation. An ES of 0.2 is generally considered 'small' (a small percentage of patients had greater improvement than the control group) and an ES of 0.8 would be considered to be 'large' (a larger percentage of the treatment group had greater improvement compared with the control group).

Table 5.2 Effect sizes in GAD	
Medication	Effect size
Pregabalin	0.50
Hydroxyzine	0.45
Venlafaxine m/r	0.42
Benzodiazepines	0.38
SSRIs	0.36
Buspirone	0.17
All	0.39

All effect sizes significant $p < 0.0001$, except for buspirone which did not reach a level of significance (Adapted from Hidalgo *et al.* 2007).

venlafaxine ranging in duration from 24 to 28 weeks. All of these studies demonstrated the efficacy of venlafaxine over placebo for most doses. In a smaller long-term study comparing escitalopram to paroxetine over 24-weeks, both drugs showed significant reduction on the primary outcome measure (change in HAMA from baseline to end point). Buspirone was examined in 24-week studies and found to be superior to placebo and equal in efficacy to clorazepate. Diazepam demonstrated superior efficacy to placebo in one 22-week study.

5.7 Relapse prevention studies

Relapse prevention studies are carried out to demonstrate maintenance of efficacy of a pharmacological agent in GAD. These studies typically involve an open label phase of treatment followed by a re-randomization of responders to drug or placebo. There have been several agents evaluated in GAD in studies with a relapse prevention design, generally showing a significant decrease in relapse for the active agent (10.9% to 42.9%) compared to placebo (39.9% to 64%) (Table 5.4).

5.8 Treatment-refractory GAD

There is relatively little systematic data concerning next-step treatments and strategies for patients with GAD refractory to standard treatment. Open label studies of aripiprazole augmentation as well as open label risperidone, ziprasidone and quetiapine have shown significant reductions in GAD symptoms (see Table 5.5). Small RCTs of olanzapine and risperidone have also demonstrated efficacy as augmentation agents for the treatment of patients with GAD who remain symptomatic despite standard anxiolytic therapy, although a larger RCT with risperidone was negative. Negative results were also found in augmentation studies of quetiapine and ziprasidone in refractory GAD, however an RCT of adjunctive pregabalin was positive.

Table 5.3 Long term studies of GAD pharmacotherapy

Drug, class and study		N	Weeks	Design	Efficacy	Comments
				Long term trials		
Azapirones						
Buspirone	Tollefson et al. (1992)	51	24	BUS (15–60 mg/day) vs. PBO	BUS > PBO	All patients GAD (DSM-III) with comorbid alcoholism
	Rickels et al. (1988)	134	24	BUS (10–40 mg/day) vs. CLO (15–40 mg/day)	BUS = CLO	DSM-III criteria
Benzodiazepines						
Diazepam	Rickels et al. (1983)	180	22	DIA (15–40 mg/day) vs. PBO (with one cross-over arm)	DIA > PBO	DSM-III criteria
SSRIs						
Escitalopram	Bielski et al. (2005)	121	24	ESC (10–20 mg/day) vs. PAR (20–50 mg/day)	ESC = PAR	
SNRIs						
Venlafaxine ER	Hackett et al. (1999)	544	24	VEN (37.5, 75, 150 mg/day) vs. PBO	VEN (150 mg/day) > VEN (37.5 mg/day) > PBO	
	Gelenberg et al. (2000)	251	28	VEN (75, 150, 225 mg/day) vs. PBO	VEN > PBO	
	Alluglander et al. (2001)	529	24	VEN (37.5, 75, 150 mg/day) vs. PBO	VEN > PBO	

Abbreviations (alphabetical): ABE = abecarnil; AGO = agomelatine; ALP = alprazolam; BUP = bupropion m/r; BUS = buspirone; CHL = chlordiazepoxide; CLO = clorazepate; DIA = diazepam; DUL = duloxetine; ESC = escitalopram; HYD = hyroxyzine; IMP = imipramine; LES = lesopitron; LOR = lorazepam; OPI = opipramol; OXA = oxazepam; PAR = paroxetine; PBO = placebo; PRO = propranolol; PRE = pregabalin; QUE = quetiapine; SER = sertraline; TIA = tiagabine; TRA = trazodone; TRI = trifluorperazine; VEN = venlafaxine ER

Table 5.4 Relapse Prevention Studies

Drug and study		Dose	N	Open	Ext	Relapse
Paroxetine	Stocchi et al. (2003)	20–50 mg/day	652	8	24	PAR: 10.9% PBO: 39.9%
Escitalopram	Allgulander et al. (2006)	20 mg/day	491	12	24–76	ESC: 19% PBO: 56%
	Bakish et al. (2006)	20 mg/day	72	12	24	ESC: 33% PBO: 64%
Pregabalin	Feltner et al. (2008)	450 mg/day	338	8	24	PGB: 42.9% PBO: 63.5%
Duloxetine	Davidson et al. (2007)	60–120 mg/day	887	26	26	DUL: 13.7% PBO: 41.9%
Quetiapine	Katzman et al. (2008)	50–300 mg/day	433	16–24	Up to 52	QUE: 10.2% PBO: 38.9%

Abbreviations (alphabetical): ESC = escitalopram; DUL = duloxetine; PAR = paroxetine; PGB = pregabalin; QUE = quetiapine

Table 5.5 Treatment refractory GAD

Drug and study	N	Weeks	Design	Efficacy	Notes
Ziprasidone					
Snyderman et al. (2005) (open label)	13	7	ZIP (20–80 mg/day)	54% response 38% remission	
Lahoff et al. (2010) (RCT)	62	8	Adjunctive or monotherapy ZIP (20–80 mg/day) vs. PBO	ZIP = PBO (adjunctive) ZIP = PBO (monotherapy)	
Pregabalin					
Weaver et al. (2009) (RCT)	353	8	Adjunctive PGB (150–600 mg/day) vs. Adjunctive PBO	PGB > PBO	
Risperidone					
Brawman-Mintzer et al. (2005)	40	5	Adjunctive RISP (0.5–1.5 mg/day) vs. PBO	RISP > PBO	Mixed primary medications
Simon et al. (2006) (open label)	30	8	Adjunctive RISP (0.25–3 mg/day)	Significant reduction on HAMA	Mixed anxiety sample (GAD: 53.3%, SAD: 23.3%, PD: 23.3%)
Padina et al. (2007)	417	4	Adjunctive RISP vs. PBO	RISP = PBO	Mixed primary medications
Olanzapine					
Pollack et al. (2006)	24	6	Adjunctive OLAN (5–20 mg/day) vs. PBO	OLAN > PBO	Primary medication fluoxetine
Quetiapine					
Simon et al. (2008)	22	8	Adjunctive QUE (25–400 mg/day) vs. PBO	QUE = PBO	Primary medication paroxetine
Katzman et al. (2008) (open label)	40	12	Adjunctive QUE (25–800 mg/day; 386 mg/day mean dose)	Significant reduction on HAMA	
Aripiprazole					
Menza et al. (2007) (open label)	9	6	Adjunctive ARI (14 mg/day—mean dose)	56% HAMA responders 89% CGI-I responders	
Hoge et al. (2008) (open label)	23	8	Adjunctive ARI (2.5–30 mg/day)	Significant reduction on HAMA and CGI-I	Mixed sample (GAD: 57%, PD: 43%)

Abbreviations (alphabetical): ABE = abecarnil; AGO = agomelatine; ALP = alprazolam; ARI = aripiprazole; ATN = atenolol; BRO = bromazepam; BUP = bupropion m/r; BUS = buspirone; CHL = chlordiazepoxide; DIA = diazepam; DUL = duloxetine; ESC = escitalopram; HYD = hyroxyzine; IMP = imipramine; LES = lesopitron; LOR = lorazepam; OPI = opipramol; OXA = oxazepam; PAR = paroxetine; PBO = placebo; PRO = propranolol; PRE = pregabalin; QUE = quetiapine; RISP = resperidone; SER = sertraline; TIA = tiagabine; TRA = trazodone; TRI = trifluorperazine ZIP = Ziprasi-done.

Cognitive behavioural therapy has been shown to be an effective treatment in GAD as compared to control conditions. Cognitive-behavioural therapy (CBT) may be a useful augmentation strategy to pharmacotherapy, although the efficacy of combining pharmacotherapy and CBT for GAD has not been well-evaluated and existing evidence is equivocal.

At this point in time there is little in the way of evidence-based strategies for treatment-resistant GAD. However, the existing data and experience suggest that augmentation with benzodiazepines, anticonvulsants, and atypical antipsychotics, as well as CBT, are reasonable strategies after consideration of their associated risk profiles.

5.9 RCTs of GAD in children

There have been very few RCTs conducted that examine the efficacy of pharmacotherapy in children and adolescents with GAD (see Table 5.6). These studies have primarily involved the SSRIs, SNRIs, and benzodiazepines. As GAD in childhood is highly co-morbid with other anxiety disorders including social phobia and separation anxiety disorder, the majority of the studies have evaluated co-morbid GAD.

Alprazolam was studied (Simeon *et al.* 1992) in a double-blind RCT in children (mean age 12.6 yrs) with DSM-III-R avoidant disorder (N = 9) and overanxious disorder (N = 21), the latter being a predecessor to DSM-IV childhood GAD. The benzodiazepine alprazolam was administered in flexible doses (1 to 4 mg/day) for 4 weeks. There were no significant differences observed between alprazolam and placebo on the primary outcome measures (Brief Psychiatric Rating Scale and Clinical Global Impression Scales).

The SSRI, sertraline (50 mg/day) was evaluated in 22 children and adolescents (mean age 11.7 yrs) with GAD in a 9-week RCT (Rynn *et al.* 2001). Sertraline-treated patients showed significant improvement over placebo beginning at week 4 on the HAMA as well as CGI scores. There was no significant differences observed between groups in the incidence of adverse events.

Flexible dose fluvoxamine (up to 300 mg/day) was evaluated in an 8-week RCT of 128 children and adolescents (mean age 11.2 yrs) with social phobia, separation anxiety, and GAD (N = 51) (Research Unit on Paediatric Psychopharmacology Anxiety Study Group 2001). At week 8, fluvoxamine was significantly more effective (p < 0.001) than placebo on the primary outcome measures (Pediatric Anxiety Rating Scale, CGI), though no disorder specific analysis was conducted. There was a significantly higher incidence of gastrointestinal side effects in the fluvoxamine-treated group over the placebo group.

Table 5.6 RCTs of GAD in children

Drug and study		Group (N)	Weeks	Design	Efficacy	Notes
Alprazolam	Simeon et al. (1992)	Over ANX (21) Sep ANX (9)	4	ALP (1–4 mg/day) vs. PBO	ALP = PBO	DSM-III-R precursors to DSM-IV GAD
Sertraline	Rynn et al. (2001)	GAD (22)	9	SER (50 mg/day) vs. PBO	SER > PBO	
Fluvoxamine	RUPP (2001)	GAD (73) SP (76) Sep ANX (76)	8	FLVX (50–300 mg/day) vs. PBO	FLVX > PBO	Patients display multiple co-morbidites
Fluoxetine	Birmaher et al. (2003)	GAD (47) Sep ANX (35) SP (41)	12	FLU (20 mg/day) vs. PBO	FLU > PBO	Patients display multiple co-morbidites
Venlafaxine m/r	Rynn et al. (2007)	GAD (320)	8	VEN (37.5–225 mg/day) vs. PBO	VEN > PBO	Pooled analysis

Group Abbreviations (alphabetical): GAD = generalized anxiety disorder; Over ANX = overanxious disorder; Sep ANX = separation anxiety; SP = social phobia.
Drug Abbreviations (alphabetical): ALP = alprazolam; FLU = fluoxetine; FLVX = fluvoxamine; SER = sertraline; VEN = venlafaxine ER

Fluoxetine (20 mg/day) was studied in a 12-week randomized control trial of children and adolescents (N = 74, mean age 11.6 yrs) with GAD, separation anxiety disorder, and/or social phobia (Birmaher *et al.* 2003). Fluoxetine (p = 0.003) was significantly better than placebo on outcome measures.

Venlafaxine m/r was evaluated in two separate randomized-controlled flexible dose (up to 225 mg/day) studies for 8 weeks in childhood and adolescent (aged 6 to 17; mean age 11.2 yrs) with GAD (Rynn *et al.* 2007). In the first study venlafaxine was significantly better than placebo on the primary outcome measure (composite score on nine items of GAD section of the Schedule for Affective Disorders and Schizophrenia for School Aged Children) though in the second study the differential efficacy of venlafaxine approached but did not achieve significance. In the pooled analysis of the 320 GAD youth, there was a significant advantage for venlafaxine m/r over placebo at end point (p < 0.001) on the primary outcome measure and response rates by CGI-I for venlafaxine 69% versus placebo 48% (p = 0.004).

The current literature on paediatric GAD suggests that the SSRIs sertraline, fluvoxamine, fluoxetine, and likely the SNRI venlafaxine are safe and efficacious; however, this was not found for the benzodiazepine alprazolam. Additional research in affected children and adolescents with these and other agents shown effective in adults is warranted.

5.10 Pharmacotherapy of GAD in the elderly

Treatment of GAD in elderly patient populations also poses its own unique challenges and therefore, treatment options must be carefully evaluated to ensure their maximum effectiveness. The age-related difficulties experienced by the elderly (declining physical health, bereavement, etc.) must also be considered in the evaluation and treatment planning of patients. Dose titration may need to be more gradual in elderly patients, because of their increased sensitivity to side effects, and the onset of therapeutic effect may require a longer period of treatment.

Although benzodiazepines have been used in treatment of older patient cohorts, elderly individuals may be particularly vulnerable to their potential adverse effects on wakefulness, cognition, and psychomotor function; consideration of downward dose adjustment or alternative strategies may be important in this population.

There are a handful of studies that have examined the effectiveness of other classes of pharmacological agents in the elderly (see Table 5.7). RCTs of the SNRIs venlafaxine and duloxetine,

Table 5.7 Pharmacotherapy of GAD in the elderly					
Drug and study		N	Weeks	Design	Efficacy	Notes
Citalopram	Lenze et al. (2005)	34	8	CIT (10–30 mg/day) vs. PBO	CIT > PBO	35% of sample concomitant lorazepam
Escitalopram	Lenze et al. (2009)	177	12	ESC (10–20 mg/day) vs. PBO	ESC = PBO (ITT)	
Venlafaxine ER	Katz et al. (2002)	136	8+	VEN (37.5–225 mg/day) vs. PBO	VEN > PBO	Pooled analysis
Pregabalin	Garcia et al. (2007)	227	8	PRE (150–600 mg/day) vs. PBO	PRE > PBO	
Quetiapine XR	Erikson et al. (2008)	450	11	QUE (50–300 mg/day) vs. PBO	QUE > PBO	Symptom improvement observed by Week 1
Duloxetine	Davidson et al. (2008)	1491	9–10	DUL (60–120 mg/day) vs. PBO	DUL > PBO	Pooled analysis
Drug abbreviations (alphabetical): CIT = citalopram; DUL = duloxetine; PRE = pregabalin; QUE = quetiapine XR; VEN = venlafaxine ER.						

the SSRI citalopram, the anticonvulsant pregabalin and the atypical antipsychotic agent, quetiapine XR have yielded positive results in older GAD patient populations. A trial of the SSRI escitalopram in an elderly population cumulative response rate for escitalopram over placebo, however, in the intent to treat analysis response rates did not significantly differ (Lenze et al., 2009).

Given the 'aging' of the population, there needs to be further studies examining the treatment of GAD in elderly individuals.

5.11 Conclusion

Our review of the pharmacotherapy of GAD gives support to a broad range of treatments from a variety of drug classes (see Table 5.8). At this point, there are no consistent predictors of treatment

Table 5.8 Evidence-based pharmacological treatment of GAD		
GAD Randomized Controlled Trials		
Drug and class	**Drug**	**Level of evidence**
SSRIs	Paroxetine	1
	Escitalopram	1
	Sertraline	1
SNRIs	Venlafaxine ER	1
	Duloxetine	1
TCAs	Imipramine	1
	Opipramol	2
Other antidepressants	Buproprion XL	2
	Agomelatine	2
Benzodiazepines	Alprazolam	1
	Bromazepam	1
	Lorazepam	1
	Diazepam	1
Antipsychotics	Quetiapine	1
Anticonvulsants	Pregabalin	1
	Tiagabine	1−
Azapirones	Buspirone	1
Antihistamines	Hydroxyzine	1
Beta-blockers	Propranolol	2−
	Atenolol	2−

− = Non-significant result.
Levels of evidence as detailed in the Canadian Clinical Practice Guidelines (Canadian Psychiatric Association 2006). Levels of evidence are ranked from 1 (best) to 4:
(1) Meta-analysis or replicated RCT that includes a placebo condition (the highest level of evidence), (2) at least one RCT with placebo or active comparison condition,
(3) uncontrolled trial with at least ten or more subjects, and (4) anecdotal reports or expert opinions.

response. As such, the initial choice of treatment needs to be based on a variety of factors including the potential efficacy of the agent, the presence of medical and or psychiatric co-morbidity, previous response to a given treatment, cost, safety, and tolerability. For most individuals treatment is generally initiated with an SSRI or SNRI, although benzodiazepines and perhaps pregabalin are reasonable alternatives in patients without significant co-morbid depression. Although currently available treatments are clearly efficacious for the treatment of GAD, there are several issues which require further attention. Clinicians require a more effective way of determining which treatments are best-suited to a given patient or patient population. Unfortunately, most of the large randomized-controlled studies in this area have been conducted in GAD patients with none or modest degrees of co-morbidity which does not reflect the typical presentation in clinical settings; systematic evaluation of the effectiveness of treatments in individuals with GAD and significant mood, anxiety, substance abuse, and other co-morbidities, as well as the young, elderly, and refractory would help inform practice.

References

Allgulander C, Hartford J, Russel J et al. (2007). Pharmacotherapy of generalized anxiety disorder: results of duloxetine treatment from a pooled analysis of three clinical trials. *Curr Med Res Opin*, **23** (6), 1245–52.

Barrett EJ. (2004). Report from ADA/APA from the Consensus Development Conference on Antipsychotic Drugs and Diabetes. Presented at the American Diabetes Association, 51st Annual Advanced Postgraduate Course, San Francisco, 6–8 February 2004.

Birmaher B, Axelson DA, Monk K et al. (2003). Fluoxetine for the treatment of childhood anxiety disorders. *J Am Acad Child Adolesc Psychiatry*, **42** (4), 415–23.

Canadian Psychiatric Association. (2006). Clinical practice guidelines: management of anxiety disorders. *Can J Psychiatry*, **51** (Suppl 2), 1S–92S.

Greenblatt DJ, Shader RI. (1974). *Benzodiazepines in Clinical Practice*. Raven Press, New York.

Hidalgo RB, Tupler LA, Davidson JRT. (2007). An effect-size analysis of pharmacologic treatments for generalized anxiety disorder. *J Psychopharmacol*, **21** (8), 864–72.

Mathew SJ, Hoffman EJ. (2009). Pharmacotherapy of generalized anxiety disorder, in: Antony MM, Stein MB (Eds). *The Oxford Handbook of Anxiety and Related Disorders*. Oxford University Press, New York, NY.

Mendels J, Krajewski TF, Huffer V, et al. (1986). Effective short-term treatment of generalized anxiety disorder with trifluoperazine. *J Am Psychiatry*, **47**, 170–4.

Napoliello MJ, Domantay AG. (1991). Buspirone: a worldwide update. *Br J Psychiatry*, **159** (Suppl 12), 40–4.

Research Unit on Pediatric Psychopharmacology Anxiety Study Group. (2001). Fluvoxamine for the treatment of anxiety disorders in children and adolescents. *N Engl J Med*, **344** (17), 1279–86.

Rynn MA, Riddle MA, Yeung PP, Kunz NR. (2007). Efficacy and safety of extended-release venlafaxine in the treatment of generalized anxiety disorder in children and adolescents: two placebo-controlled trials. *Am J Psychiatry*, **164** (2), 290–300.

Rynn MA, Siqueland L, Rickels K. (2001). Placebo-controlled trial of sertraline in the treatment of children with generalized anxiety disorder. *Am J Psychiatry*, **158**, 2008–14.

Seeman P. (2002). Atypical antipsychotics: mechanism of action. *Can Psychiatry*, **47** (1), 27–38.

Simeon JG, Ferguson BH, Knott V et al. (1992). Clinical, cognitive and neurophysiological effects of alprazolam in children and adolescents with overanxious and avoidant disorder. *J Am Acad Child Adolesc Psychiatry*, **31** (1), 29–33.

Van Ameringen M, Mancini C, Patterson B, Simpson W, Truong C. (2009). The pharmacotherapy of generalized anxiety disorder, in: *APPI Textbook of Anxiety Disorders*, Second Edition. American Psychiatric Publishing Inc., Washington DC, pp. 193–218.

Zavoianu M, Luchian A, Tudor C et al. (2009). Efficacy of trazodone in patients diagnosed with generalized anxiety disorder and benzodiazepine dependence. *European Neuropsychopharmacol*, **19**, Suppl 3, S617–8.

Chapter 6

Psychotherapy

Beth Patterson, Michael Van Ameringen,
and Mark H. Pollack

Key points

- Individual or group cognitive behavioural therapy (CBT)
  has demonstrated consistent efficacy in the treatment of
  generalized anxiety disorder (GAD).
- Key components of CBT include psychoeducation,
  breathing retraining, progressive muscle relaxation,
  cognitive restructuring, and graded exposure.

6.1 Early treatment modalities

Psychotherapy techniques for generalized anxiety disorder (GAD)
have evolved considerably over the past two decades in keeping with
changes in the diagnostic nomenclature. Early psychotherapeutic
techniques for GAD were aimed at treating general anxious arousal
and employed strategies designed to treat the pervasive experience
of anxiety rather than the specific processes behind the development
and maintenance of the disorder (Robichaud and Dugas 2008). These
early strategies included exposure to target phobic avoidance, as well
as anxiety management techniques such as imagery rehearsal to treat
the somatic symptoms. Another intervention, stimulus control involves
training the individual to delay the worry and focus on the current
moment's experience, then scheduling a future time to engage in the
worry. This was one of the few techniques designed specifically for
GAD. Relaxation techniques have been a mainstay in the treatment
of GAD and have been used in various forms as coping strategies in
response to anxiety cues. Applied relaxation, developed by Öst (Öst
1987) for the treatment of phobias, is a technique that has been
adapted for use in GAD and was a primary component of early psychotherapeutic treatment. It involves having individuals develop 20 to
30 second relaxation strategies for use in real-life anxiety-provoking
situations. Applied relaxation technique training begins with progressive muscle relaxation (where various muscle groups are tensed and
relaxed) and progresses to rapid relaxation in 20 to 30 seconds.

Diaphragmatic breathing is another technique commonly incorporated into relaxation training to decrease somatic arousal.

6.2 Cognitive behavioural therapy (CBT)

Cognitive therapy has been a key component of both early and more recent GAD psychosocial treatment programmes. General cognitive strategies such as self-monitoring, identifying faulty thinking patterns, and generating alternative, more realistic thoughts are typically utilized in CBT for GAD, with specific emphasis on decatastrophizing and challenging thoughts with probability estimations (Box 6.1). CBT for GAD has been shown to be effective in both individual and group formats. A recent report suggests that CBT for GAD may also be effective using a clinician-assisted, internet-based treatment modality (Titov *et al.* 2009). Although psychodynamic and supportive treatments (either active or inactive) continue to be used in the treatment of GAD, they lack the positive empirical evidence which supports the use of CBT (Hunot *et al.* 2008).

Several meta-analytic literature reviews have examined CBT for GAD; CBT has been found to be consistently superior when compared to wait-list controls or treatment as usual (Hunot *et al.* 2008). Effect sizes have ranged from 0.51 to 2.48 (moderate to large). Covin and colleagues (Covin *et al.* 2008) recently conducted a meta-analysis of CBT in terms of its ability to treat pathological worry, the hallmark symptom of GAD. The overall effect size (ES)[*] was large (1.15) in the between groups analysis.

Box 6.1 Typical components of CBT for GAD
Psychoeducation: Aetiology, course, and treatment of GAD; rationale and efficacy of CBT
Breathing retraining: Diaphragmatic breathing to help reduce physical symptoms
Progressive muscle relaxation: To help reduce physical symptoms
Cognitive restructuring: To address maladaptive worry and develop new coping strategies
Graded exposure: Both *in vivo* and *in vitro* exposure are used to help patients practice coping skills in situations involving worry and anxiety

[*] Effect size (ES) is a measure of the magnitude of treatment effect across several studies as compared to a control treatment. It is statistical method frequently used in meta-analyses which summarizes several studies into a single estimate after a standard measure of effect has been calculated for each study. The ES is roughly the difference between the mean values of the two groups, divided by the standard deviation. An ES of 0.2 is generally considered 'small' (a small percentage of patients had greater improvement than the control group) and an ES of 0.8 would be considered to be 'large' (a larger percentage of the treatment group had greater improvement compared with the control group).

An additional weighted analysis indicated that although all results were significant, the effect was strongest in younger adults (1.69) versus older adults (0.82), suggesting decreased efficacy of CBT as individuals age. Although CBT for GAD has apparent efficacy, the rate of remission is quite modest when compared to that achieved by CBT for other anxiety disorders with more phobic elements. In a meta-analysis conducted by Hofmann and Smits (2008), the effect sizes for GAD (0.57 and 0.44) were of the lowest of the anxiety disorders (ES for OCD ranged from 0.74 to 2.08). Remission rates achieved by CBT in GAD have been reported to be roughly 50% at 6-month follow-up, and 30% to 40% recovered at 3- to 8-yr follow-up (Flint 2005).

The efficacy of CBT as compared to pharmacotherapy for GAD has also been examined meta-analytically. Both treatments were found to be equal in efficacy, although CBT had lower drop-out rate (Mitte 2005).

6.3 **CBT in special populations**

The efficacy of CBT for GAD has been examined in elderly populations, in whom it has been found to be more effective than wait-list control. However the response rates (28% to 45%) were lower than those found in studies of younger adults, and rates of remission even lower still (3% to 22%). In addition, CBT in the elderly was reported no more effective than a discussion group and less effective than supportive counselling (Flint 2005). There has been some speculation that CBT in the elderly is more effective when delivered on an individual basis as opposed to group therapy; however, further research is required to provide therapists with clear guidance on this issue.

In children and adolescents with GAD, psychological treatment is multifaceted. CBT is generally simpler and more concrete and the specific approach modified based on the needs of the individual. The treatment of children and adolescents often involves additional interventions such as social skills training and problem-solving training to assist patients with their anxiety difficulties. Further, provision of psychoeducation for parents, other family members, and teachers may also be incorporated into treatment; most CBT programmes aimed at this population also actively involve the families of patients in the treatment process. In randomized, placebo-controlled investigations of CBT conducted to date, the paediatric populations have included a mixture of anxiety disorders, including GAD (or overanxious disorder), and employed general CBT protocols, such as Kendall's 'Coping Cat' programme (Kendell 1994). Nevertheless, the efficacy of CBT in childhood anxiety disorders overall has been quite positive with remission rates of 68.9% (compared with 12.9% in wait-list control groups) (In-Albon and Schneider 2007). A recent meta-analysis also demonstrated very large effect sizes for CBT in childhood/adolescent anxiety disorders (0.86 in CBT conditions versus 0.12 in wait-list controls) (In-Albon and Schneider 2007). CBT in children and adolescents appears to be effective when delivered in either a group or individual format.

6.4 **Treatment protocols**

Recent CBT treatments have become more specific for GAD in the hopes that treating the underlying processes will result in improved treatment outcomes. There are several treatment approaches utilized in these protocols, the first two of which have been empirically evaluated:

1. Cognitive avoidance (Borkovec 2006)
2. Intolerance of uncertainty (IU) (Dugas and Robichaud 2007)
3. Metacognitive therapy (Wells 2009).

6.5 **Cognitive avoidance treatment model**

In the cognitive avoidance model, worry is conceptualized as a cognitive avoidance strategy in terms of: (a) its suppression of anxious arousal, (b) its function as an attempt to prevent or prepare for the future, and (c) its role in distracting from more present-moment emotional concerns by focusing on superficial events. This treatment protocol emphasizes focus on the 'present-moment' as opposed to the past or future-oriented thinking characteristic of GAD and subsequently exposes patients to the imagery and physiological arousal they have been avoiding.

There are four primary components of this treatment model:

1. *Awareness and self-monitoring* to help patients identify and recognize the triggers of their anxiety and their maladaptive reactions to these triggers. Patients learn to become more aware of shifts in their anxiety so that they can intervene with new coping skills at the very beginning of an anxious episode.
2. *Relaxation training* where patients are taught to use relaxation strategies in every day situations as well as in anxiety situations to learn to feel calm in the present-moment. The techniques include progressive muscle relaxation, applied relaxation, and breathing retraining.
3. *Cognitive therapy*. In this phase of treatment, patients are encouraged to keep a worry outcome diary. Daily worries and their feared outcomes are recorded, then reviewed each evening. For any worries whose outcome is known once reviewed, patients record their ability to cope with the outcome

and rate if they coped better or worse than predicted. Most patients find that the outcome was not as bad as anticipated and that they coped better than anticipated. Traditional methods of replacing inaccurate thoughts with more realistic appraisals are used; however in this model, the end goal of cognitive therapy is that individuals will learn to live free of expectations for the future. This is quite different than previous models where faulty or maladaptive thought patterns are identified and corrected. According to Borkevec, living without expectations enables an individual with GAD to more accurately appraise present situations without the bias imposed by a preconception or prediction, since individuals tend to process information based on pre-existing beliefs. Patients are encouraged to practise entering novel situations with minimum expectations about what the present moment will bring (Borkovec 2006).

4. *Imagery rehearsal of coping strategies* in response to imagery of an anxiety-provoking situation. Patients are encouraged to visualize an anxiety-inducing scene, experience the anxiety, and utilize relaxation techniques to return to a relaxed state. This is done repeatedly, both in session and at home. Patients are thus exposed to the types of imagery and physiological arousal they have been avoiding.

The cognitive avoidance model has been evaluated in several controlled trials and has been found to be superior compared to non-directive treatment, and equal in efficacy to behaviour therapy and cognitive therapy. Despite resulting in significant improvement from baseline, high end-state functioning was only achieved in about half of the patients treated (Borkovec and Costello 1993; Borkovec *et al.* 2002).

6.6 Intolerance of uncertainty treatment model

Developed by Dugas and colleagues, the central premise of this model is the idea that individuals with GAD are much more intolerant of uncertainty in day-to-day life as compared to people without the disorder. IU describes a characteristic that 'results from a set of negative beliefs about uncertainty and its implications' (Dugas and Robichaud 2007). When faced with uncertainty, individuals with GAD will respond with worry in an attempt to think about and plan for any eventuality (e.g. If this happens, then I will respond by . . .) (Robichaud and Dugas 2008). Considering that uncertainty is rampant in daily life, an individual with GAD is frequently plagued by worry such that it becomes excessive and uncontrolled. In order to help patients to become more tolerant of uncertainty in daily life, the IU model teaches patients to separate their worry into two categories:

those that will respond to problem-solving and those that will not (Covin *et al.* 2008). Previous GAD treatment protocols have incorporated probability estimation as a key technique in helping people judge how realistic the worry is and to judge whether or not to discard the worry. In the IU treatment protocol, patients are expected to worry and to eventually habituate to the idea of living with uncertainty. As long as the possibility of a catastrophic outcome exists, however slim, Dugas and colleagues assert that worry will be maintained in an individual with GAD unless their ability to tolerate uncertainty is addressed. Neuroimaging data have recently linked insula hyperactivity in anxiety disorders to an individual's IU when viewing ambiguous stimuli, lending support to the underlying focus of this treatment intervention (Simmons *et al*, 2008). Each component of the treatment protocol was substantiated by clinical and non-clinical research based on the cognitive model of GAD (Robichaud and Dugas 2008).

The IU protocol is comprised of six treatment modules:

1. *Psychoeducation and worry awareness training*: Principles of CBT are introduced, the diagnosis of GAD is explained, including the IU model of interpreting the symptoms of GAD. Worry awareness training is also included in this module, where the patient's own worries are identified and monitored.

2. *The recognition of uncertainty and behavioural exposure*: In this module, IU is reviewed in terms of its role in the development and maintenance of excessive worry and anxiety. Patients begin to recognize and deal with uncertainty in their day-to-day lives using behavioural exposure. Behavioural experiments are ranked in order of difficulty and conducted in a progressive manner (i.e. experiments related to patients' major worry themes are conducted last). Experiments could include activities such as not checking low-priority e-mails or making minor decisions without seeking reassurance. Patients are asked to conduct at least one experiment per week where they attempt to tolerate uncertainty in situations. The exposure is designed to assist patients in the developing new strategies to deal with uncertainty.

3. *Re-evaluation of the usefulness of worry*: Positive beliefs concerning the usefulness of worry are acknowledged and challenged. Generally, the beliefs fall into several main categories: that worry is helpful in finding solutions to problems; that worry serves as a motivating function, ensuring that tasks will get completed; that worry can protect from negative emotions; that worry can prevent negative outcomes; and that worry is a positive personality trait. This module is very important to the success of the treatment protocol as patients need to have accurate appraisals of whether or not their worry is beneficial in order to tackle any ambivalence experienced in treatment.

4. *Training in problem solving:* In the first module, patients are taught to distinguish between worries that deal with current problems and worries about hypothetical situations. A problem-solving approach is used for current, actual problems. Instruction on how to improve patients' problem orientation, that is changing their negative beliefs about problems as well as their own problem-solving ability. Patients are encouraged to examine relative threat of problems on a dimensional level as opposed to a categorical level and to find the opportunity within a given situation to facilitate problem solving. These steps are practised both in session and in between visits. Problem solving can be conceptualized as a more active approach to dealing with difficulties as opposed to worry where problems are thought about but not solved.

5. *Imaginal exposure:* This technique is used for dealing with hypothetical problems or situations. The module is based upon research evidence indicating that worry takes the form of verbal-linguistic thoughts instead of mental images, which decreases physiological arousal. Patients are encouraged to actively visualize catastrophic outcomes by writing a detailed account in story format, including as much sensory and visual detail as possible. Patients then use this script to conduct daily imaginal exposures until the anxiety and distress is dampened.

6. *Relapse prevention:* Patients are encouraged to continue using the skills they have learned to maintain progress long after the cessation of treatment. This modules includes tips for daily maintenance and the identification of at-risk situations as well as preparation for at-risk situations.

The IU protocol does not include a relaxation module to directly address the somatic symptoms of worry. These symptoms are expected to improve as worry is dampened through the development of a greater tolerance for uncertainty. This protocol has been well-evaluated in the literature. It has been consistently shown to be superior to wait-list control, on all measures of symptom severity following treatment with roughly two-thirds of patients responding to treatment administered in either group or individual formats. At 1-yr follow-up 58% of patients who had been treated with individual therapy and 66% of patients treated in a group format had maintained their gains of high end state functioning (Robichaud and Dugas 2008). In a study of 65 adults with GAD comparing CBT (with IU) to applied relaxation (AR), CBT was significantly superior to waitlist control (WL) (but AR = WL). CBT was not found to be significantly superior to AR at endpoint, however only CBT led to greater improvement over time. At the post-treatment time point, remission was found in 70% treated with CBT using IU versus 55% treated with applied relaxation, although the difference between treatments was not significant (Dugas *et al.* 2010).

6.7 **Metacognitive therapy**

A third psychological disorder-specific treatment approach is meta-cognitive therapy (Wells 2009). The focus of this treatment is the patients' beliefs about worry, not the worries themselves. This treatment model is based on the assertion that worry in GAD arises from the positive and negative beliefs an individual has about worry. Positive beliefs include the idea that worry is useful to assist with successful resolution of the problem at hand and that worry will end once the difficulty is resolved. Worry in GAD occurs with the addition of negative beliefs about worry such as, 'worry is dangerous or hard to control' and this leads to worry about worrying ('meta-worry'). Achieving a resolution to a problem becomes impossible as the worry is so cyclical in nature. The worry then becomes excessive and chronic.

The protocol uses five key components to modify patients' beliefs about worry:

1. *Case formulation*: The patient's worries are identified, classified, and given a pictorial representation. Type I worries are those concerning day-to-day life events; Type II worries are meta-worries. The emotional, behavioural, and cognitive consequences of meta-worry for the patient are also identified in this step.

2. *Socialization to treatment*: In this step, the model developed in the first module is examined in terms of the ineffectiveness of the patient's current coping strategies. Patients are encouraged to look towards the end goal of changing their beliefs about worry.

3. *Modifying negative beliefs*: This is accomplished using cognitive behavioural strategies. For example, evidence supporting and disconfirming specific beliefs is examined; patients are encouraged either to delay engaging in the worry process or to deliberately activate it with worry to demonstrate that worry can be controlled.

4. *Modifying beliefs concerning the danger of worry*: Further cognitive and behavioural strategies are used to address the patient's negative beliefs about worry (i.e. that worry is dangerous, or harmful) 'danger metacognitions'. Patients are asked to rate the strength of these metacognitions or beliefs (0 = no strength to 10 = extremely strong) and the CBT strategies are continued until a rating of 0 is achieved.

5. *Modifying positive beliefs about worry*: In this final stage, specific cognitive strategies are used including a mismatch technique where patients are instructed to record the disparity between feared and actual outcomes in order to highlight that their worry may not be particularly useful or accurate. In addition,

worry modulation experiments are conducted where patients alternate days of either increasing or decreasing their worry. They are instructed to document whether positive outcomes occur on the days with increased worry.

This treatment protocol does not specifically address somatic symptoms of anxiety as it is expected that these symptoms will improve as negative and positive worry appraisal are modified. In addition, the cognitive strategies used in metacognitive therapy do not challenge the distortions in the content of Type I (day to day) worry as is common in many CBT protocols. Instead, Wells (2009) asserts that by effectively treating meta-worry (Type II worry) the underlying processes behind the development and maintenance of GAD are ameliorated. This treatment protocol has been evaluated in an open trial in a small sample of 10 patients where 87.5% of patients met criteria for meaningful change at post-treatment (75% at follow-up) (Wells and King 2006).

6.8 Summary

There is a general consensus that GAD is one of the most difficult anxiety disorders to treat, despite being one of the most commonly seen psychiatric disorders in general practice. CBT consistently produces evidence in support of its use in GAD and has demonstrated superiority to both no-treatment conditions as well as non-directive counselling. The efficacy of CBT in GAD following completion may persist over time to a greater degree than that seen with pharmacotherapy, though long-term studies are needed to provide firm conclusions in this regard. Although these techniques appear to be effective in treating symptoms of GAD, they do not seem to produce as significant changes as seen in other anxiety disorders (Hofmann and Smits 2008). Furthermore, the efficacy of GAD seems to be less effective in elderly GAD patients. Empirically evaluated, disorder-specific treatment protocols including the cognitive avoidance model and the IU model have been valuable additions to the GAD treatment armamentarium.

References

Borkovec TD. (2006). Applied relaxation and cognitive therapy for pathological worry and generalized anxiety disorder, in: Davey, GC, Wells A (Eds). *Worry and It's Psychological Disorders: Theory, Assessment and Treatment*. John Wiley & Sons, Hoboken, NJ, pp. 274–87.

Borkovec TD, Costello E. (1993). Efficacy of applied relaxation and cognitive behavioral therapy in the treatment of generalized anxiety disorder. *J Consult Clin Psychol*, **61** (4), 611–9.

Borkovec TD, Newman MG, Pincus AL, Lytle R. (2002). A component analysis of cognitve behavioral therapy for generalized anxiety disorder and the role of interpersonal problems. *J Consult Clin Psychol*, **70** (2), 288–98.

Covin R, Ouimet AJ, Seeds PM, Dozois DJA. (2008). A meta-analysis of CBT for pathological worry among clients with GAD. *J Anx Disord*, **22** (1), 108–16.

Dugas MJ, Robichaud M. (2007). *The Cognitive-Behavioral Treatment of Generalized Anxiety Disorder: From Science to Practice.* Routledge, New York.

Dugas MJ, Brillon P, Savard P, et al. (2010). A randomized clinical trial of cognitive behavioral therapy and applied relaxation for adults with generalized anxiety disorder. *Behav Ther*, **41**, 46–58.

Flint AJ. (2005). Generalised anxiety disorder in elderly patients: epidemiology, diagnosis and treatment options. *Drugs Aging*, **22** (2), 101–14.

Hofmann SG, Smits JAJ. (2008). Cognitive behavioral therapy for adult anxiety disorders: A meta-analysis of placebo-controlled trials. *J Clin Psychiatry*, **69** (4), 621–32.

Hunot V, Churchill R, Teixeira V, Silva de Lima M. (2008). Psychological therapies for generalised anxiety disorder (Review). *The Cochrane Database Syst Rev*, (4), 1–75.

In-Albon T, Schneider S. (2007). Psychotherapy of childhood anxiety disorders: a meta-analysis. *Psychother Psychosomatics*, **76** (1), 15–24.

Kendall PC. (1994). Treating anxiety disorder in children: results of a randomized clinical trial. *J Consult Clin Psychol*, **62** (1), 100–10.

Mitte K. (2005). Meta-analysis of cognitive-behavioral treatments for generalized anxiety disorder: a comparison with pharmacotherapy. *Psychol Bull*, **131** (5), 785–95.

Ost LG. (1987). Applied relaxation: description of a coping technique and review of controlled studies. *Behav Res Ther*, **25** (5), 397–409.

Robichaud M, Dugas MJ. (2008). Psychological treatment of generalized anxiety disorder, in: Antony MM, Stein MB (Eds). *Oxford Handbook of Anxiety and Related Disorders.* Oxford University Press, New York, pp. 364–75.

Simmons A, Matthews SC, Paulus MP, Stein MB. (2008). Intolerance of uncertainty correlates with insula activation during affective ambiguity. *Neurosci Lett*, **430** (2), 92–7.

Titov N, Andrews G, Robinson E et al. (2009). Clinician-assisted internet-based treatment is effective for generalized anxiety disorder: randomized controlled trial. *Aus NZ J of Psychiatry*, **43**, 905–12.

Wells A. (2009). *Metacognitive Therapy for Anxiety and Depression.* The Guildford Press, New York, NY.

Wells A, King P. (2006). Metacognitve therapy for generalized anxiety disorder: an open trial. *J Behav Ther Exp Psychiatry*, **37** (3), 206–12.

Recommended resources for CBT

Borkovec TD. (2006). Applied relaxation and cognitive therapy for pathological worry and generalized anxiety disorder, in: Davey GC, Wells A (Eds). *Worry and It's Psychological Disorders: Theory, Assessment and Treatment.* John Wiley & Sons, Hoboken, NJ, pp. 274–87.

Craske MG, Barlow DH, O'Leary TA. (1992). *Mastery of Your Anxiety and Worry: Client Workbook.* Graywind Publications Inc, USA.

Dugas MJ, Robichard M. (2007). *The Cognitive-Behavioral Treatment of Generalized Anxiety Disorder: From Science to Practice.* Routledge, New York, NY.

Hazlett-Stevens H. (2008). *Psychological Approaches to Generalized Anxiety Disorder: A Clinician's Guide to Assessment and Treatment.* Springer, New York, NY.

Rugh JL, Sanderson WC. (2004). *Treating Generalized Anxiety Disorder: Evidence-Based Strategies, Tools, and Techniques.* The Guilford Press, New York, NY.

Wells A. (2009) *Metacognitive Therapy for Anxiety and Depression.* The Guilford Press, New York, NY.

Zinbarg RE, Craske MG, Barlow DH. (1993). *Mastery of Your Anxiety and Worry: Therapist Guide.* Oxford University Press, New York, NY.

Chapter 7

Clinical management

Michael Van Ameringen and Mark H. Pollack

Key points

- Diagnosis of generalized anxiety disorder (GAD) should involve screening for the presence of medical or other psychiatric conditions.
- Primary GAD treatment strategy involves either pharmacological or psychological treatment.
- End goal of treatment is remission or loss of diagnostic status without functional impairment.
- Pharmacological treatment should be maintained 12 to 24 months after achieving remission.
- Treatment choices and strategies need to be modified in special populations (children, the elderly, and pregnant and breastfeeding women).

7.1 Initial assessment of patients with anxiety

Individuals suffering from GAD often present with psychological symptoms such as complaints of anxiety, stress, or 'bad nerves'. Screening questions such as 'Have you been having any problems with excessive stress, worry, or anxiety?' may be useful in assessing GAD symptoms (see Table 7.1). If anxiety symptoms are endorsed, these symptoms should be explored in more detail to include the onset of the anxiety symptoms, associations with life events or trauma, the nature of the anxiety (i.e. worry, avoidance, or obsession), and the impact it has had on the current functioning of the patient.

Other potential causes of the anxiety symptoms need to be ruled out in the assessment of patients with GAD. These include an underlying medical condition, symptoms secondary to a medication, other psychiatric conditions such as depression, substance use or abuse, somatoform disorders, or psychotic disorders. The presence of medical or other psychiatric conditions does not preclude the diagnosis of an anxiety disorder, since patients with anxiety disorders

Table 7.1 Screening questions for GAD

- Are you a worrier by nature?
- Do people who know you see you as a worry wart?
- Are your worries so hard to control that they take over your life?
- Do you find yourself worrying a lot about bad things that might happen in the future?
- Do you worry a lot about day-to-day activities or getting things done?
- Does the worry prevent you from sleeping or interfere with your day-to-day functioning?
- When you are worrying do you experience muscle tension, tiredness, headaches, or stomach upset?

frequently have co-morbid conditions. Furthermore, anxiety disorders are more common in patients with a number of medical and psychiatric conditions (see Chapter 3).

The presence of certain risk factors including a family history of an anxiety disorder, a personal history of stressful or traumatic life event, and a childhood onset of anxiety symptoms increases the possibility of a GAD diagnosis. Although GAD can begin in early adulthood, recognition and diagnosis may be delayed. New onset of anxiety symptoms may begin after the age of 45, without a childhood history of significant shyness, separation anxiety, or anxiety disorder; however, *de novo* emergence of anxiety symptoms later in life without a personal or family history of anxiety or precipitant environmental stressors suggests additional scrutiny should be given to potential medical disorders which may be contributing to or be responsible for the emergent anxiety. The psychiatric history of a patient presenting with GAD symptoms should include a review of systems, prescribed medications including over-the-counter agents, alcohol use, caffeine intake, and drug use or abuse. Furthermore, a targeted physical evaluation should focus on the locus of prominent somatic symptoms (e.g. cardiovascular). The appropriate laboratory investigations will follow from the findings of a history that focuses on general medical conditions that can mimic anxiety disorders. Table 7.2 lists potential investigations which might be considered depending on the patient's specific symptomatic presentation (Canadian Psychiatric Association, 2006).

Table 7.2 Laboratory investigations to assess common concurrent medical causes of anxiety

• Complete blood count	• Liver function tests
• Lipid profile	• Urinalysis
• Thyroid screen	• Electrocardiogram
• Chemistry profile including glucose	• Toxicology screen

7.2 **When to treat**

Anxiety symptoms can be part of everyday life and exist on a continuum. Milder forms of anxiety, including anxiety of recent onset, will often improve without any specific intervention, particularly if the anxiety is triggered by a stressful life event. In these types of situations, it is appropriate to consider 'watchful waiting'. However, in many cases, patients may have been experiencing difficulty for extended periods of time before seeking care in the general medical or mental health setting, and thus require more active intervention. The need for anxiety treatment is determined by the severity and persistence of symptoms, the presence of co-morbid psychiatric or physical illness, the level of disability and impact on social functioning, and the use of concomitant medication. Intervention for anxiety-related symptoms should be strongly considered when patients experience considerable distress or impaired function. The chronicity and disability associated with symptoms reaching diagnostic threshold argue for the importance of treatment in affected individuals.

7.3 **Choice of treatment**

7.3.1 **Overview of treatment**

All GAD patients require education about their disorder that includes a discussion of the risks and benefits of treatment choices and the potential course of illness. Self-help reading materials and websites which describe evidence-based treatment strategies may be beneficial (see Chapter 8). Information from these sources helps facilitate patients in decision making with regard to effective treatments, common side effects, probable duration of treatment and what to except from treatment.

The primary treatment choices for GAD include both pharmacological and psychological treatment modalities that are reviewed in Chapters 5 and 6. A number of factors come into play when choosing the right treatment for an individual patient. Key to this decision is a patient's preference and the availability of treatment resources. In many areas, the availability of individuals trained to provide empirically based psychosocial treatments is rather limited. Other factors that must be taken into consideration include the presence of co-morbid psychiatric and medical conditions, prior treatment response, cost of treatment, patient motivation, the presence of cognitive impairment (which will limit the use of cognitive behavioural treatment), and the skills and expertise of the treating clinician.

7.3.2 **Duration of treatment**

The goal of treatment is to attain remission: elimination of significant symptoms, dysfunction, and disability. The initial treatment response for onset of symptom relief often takes 4 to 8 weeks (sometimes sooner for treatment with benzodiazepines and pregabalin and longer for cognitive behavioural therapy [CBT]) and a complete treatment response (remission) can sometimes be seen after 12 to 16 weeks. When symptomatic remission is achieved, pharmacological treatment and follow-up should be maintained for at least an additional 12 to 24 months, as longer treatment has been associated with the prevention of relapse and further symptom improvement. Some patients, however, will need ongoing maintenance therapy. Medication needs to be tapered down slowly (e.g. 10 mg paroxetine or 37.5 to 75 mg venlafaxine every 1 to 4 weeks) to minimize emergent withdrawal symptomatology or rebound; for some patients the discontinuation process may extend over a period of many months. During the medication taper period patients should be monitored for the re-emergence of anxiety symptoms. Should this occur, the reinstatement of the maintenance medication dose may be required; initiation of CBT prior to the onset or during the taper process may be helpful in managing the withdrawal symptoms and giving the patients alternative strategies to deal with their anxiety symptoms. During the medication taper phase, the clinician should be alert to the potential for withdrawal symptoms or re-emergent anxiety which may indicate the need for a slower and more gradual dose titration.

7.3.3 **Dosing**

Medications should be initiated at a low dose (e.g. 5 mg/day escitalopram, 0.25 mg clonazepam/od-bid) in order to minimize emergent side effects (e.g. sedation with benzodiazepines or exacerbation of anxiety with antidepressants). Patients should typically be seen within 1 to 2 weeks after the initiation of treatment to assess tolerability of the medication, and symptomatic progress, and address any issues that may interfere with adherence. Medication increases can occur gradually at 1- to 2-week intervals. With this dose titration schedule, patients should be within the recommended therapeutic dose range by 4 to 6 weeks after treatment initiation. Patients may start to experience some improvement in symptoms with benzodiazepines, anticonvulsants, or atypical antipsychotics within the first week or two of treatment. Although response to antidepressants may take at least 3 to 4 weeks, substantial benefit may occur after 4 to 8 weeks at a therapeutic dose and treatment gains may continue to accrue for 6 to 12 months or longer. During the first 6 weeks of treatment patients should typically be re-assessed at 1- to 2-week intervals as dosages are adjusted then at monthly or bi-monthly intervals thereafter, although the necessary frequency of visits will vary with an individual patient (Table 7.3).

For patients who initiate CBT, therapy sessions usually occur weekly for about 12 to 20 weeks with a subsequent follow-up appointment 4 weeks later. Some patients also may benefit from booster sessions at monthly intervals for 2 to 3 months after the completion of their CBT therapy sessions.

Table 7.3 Medication doses in GAD			
Drug and class	Starting dose (mg/day)	Therapeutic dose range (mg/day)	Dosing frequency
Selective serotonin re-uptake inhibitor (SSRIs)			
Escitalopram	5	10–20	OD
Paroxetine	10	20–60	OD
Sertraline	25	50–200	OD
Fluoxetine	10	20–80	OD
Fluvoxamine	50	100–300	OD
Citalopram	10	20–60	OD
Selective serotonin noradrenaline re-uptake inhibitor (SNRIs)			
Venlafaxine ER	37.5	75–225	OD–BID
Duloxetine	30	60–120	OD
Tricyclic antidepressants (TCAs)			
Imipramine	25	75–200	OD
Clomipramine	25	75–250	OD
Nortriptyline	25	100–200	OD
Desipramine	25	100–200	OD
Opipramol	50	50–200	OD
Other antidepressants			
Buproprion XL	150	150–300	OD
Agomelatine	25	25–50	OD
Benzodiazepines			
Alprazolam	0.25	0.25–4	TID–QID
Bromazepam	6	6–30	BID
Chlordiazepoxide	15	15–100	TID–QID
Clorazepate	15	15–60	BID–TID
Oxazepam	30	30–120	TID–QID
Diazepam	2.5	2.5–40	BID
Lorazepam	0.5	1–8	TID–QID
Clonazepam	0.25	1–4	BID
Azapirones			
Buspirone	10	10–60	BID–TID

Table 7.3 (Contd.)			
Drug and class	Starting dose (mg/day)	Therapeutic dose range (mg/day)	Dosing frequency
Anticonvulsants			
Pregabalin	25	150–600	BID–TID
Typical antipsychotics			
Trifluoperazine	2	2–6	OD
Atypical antipsychotics			
Quetiapine	25	50–300	OD
Risperidone	0.25	0.5–3	OD
Olanzapine	2.5	2.5–10	OD
Aripiprazole	2	2–15	OD
Ziprasidone	20	20–80	OD
Antihistamines			
Hydroxyzine	25	25–75	TID

7.4 Safety and adverse events

Please see Chapter 5 for details on safety and adverse events.

7.5 Assessing response to treatment

Treatment response is determined by assessing the degree of symptom reduction of the core symptoms of GAD (i.e. worry, tension, irritability, sleep disturbance, concentration difficulties, restlessness, fatigue). Changes in the symptoms of the co-morbid psychiatric conditions as well as social and occupational functional impairment should also be routinely monitored. Treatment progress can be accurately measured through the use of rating scales either clinician administered (such as the Hamilton Anxiety Rating Scale (HAMA)) or self-report (see Appendix for list). Although rating scales may be time consuming for both clinicians and patients, they can be useful tools for assessing treatment response over a variety of domains. A positive response to a given GAD treatment is usually defined as a 50% reduction in symptoms on the HAMA. The end goal of treatment ie., remission is typically defined as being virtually free of all symptoms with loss of diagnostic status and no impairment noted in the areas of social or occupational functioning. In clinical trials and research studies of GAD treatment, remission is defined as a HAMA score ≤ 7.

7.6 Treatment non-response

There is relatively little systematic data to inform the development of an evidence-based algorithm for non- or incomplete treatment response in GAD. Non-response, or lack of an adequate treatment response, can be determined after patients have received an adequate dose and duration (8 to 12 weeks at an optimal dose) of a given treatment. However, it may sometimes be necessary to intervene earlier for patients in marked distress or to encourage their continued adherence to treatment. The benefits of dose escalation after achieving an initial target dose are unclear as several fixed dose studies have shown little differences between dose levels. Treatment compliance should also be assessed before switching to or augmenting with another treatment. If a GAD patient has a non-response or is unable to tolerate a first-line agent, it is reasonable to consider another first-line agent (Table 7.4) (Baldwin et al., 2005).

Some clinicians would advocate switching to another agent in the case of intolerability or complete non-response to the first agent, and augmenting in the event of partial response to the initial treatment. There is, however, little systematic data addressing the relative merits of either of these approaches. In the case of a switch, the clinician could choose an agent from the same drug class or an agent with different characteristics and mechanism of action, such as a switch from an SSRI to an SNRI. For patients with multiple non-responsive trials, it is always worth reassessing the diagnosis (e.g. does the patient have co-morbid bipolar rather than unipolar disorder that may be affecting the response to an antidepressant?) and consideration

Table 7.4 Selecting a GAD treatment agent		
	Pure GAD	**GAD + Co-morbidity (i.e. depression)**
First-line agents	SSRIs	SSRIs
	SNRIs	SNRIs
	Pregabalin	
	Benzodiazepines	
Second-line agents	TCAs	TCAs
	Other antidepressants	Other antidepressants
	Atypical antipsychotics	
	Buspirone	
	Hydroxyzine	

Note: Choice of agents governed by co-morbidity and efficacy of agent in GAD + co-morbid condition (i.e. obsessive compulsive disorder co-morbidity + GAD—use SSRI first; social phobia co-morbidity + GAD use SSRI/SNRI first).

whether other relevant factors such as occult substance abuse or medical illness may be affecting treatment response. The use of CBT, if available, as an alternative or augmentation strategy should be considered as an option, as should consultation with a specialist in anxiety. See one proposed treatment algorithm (Figure 7.1).

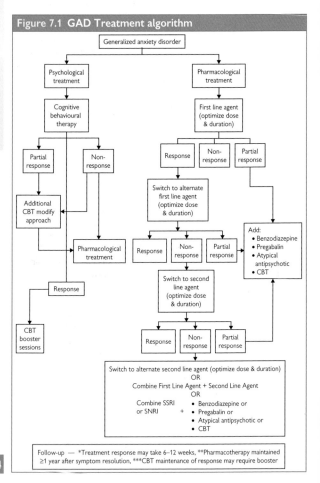

Figure 7.1 GAD Treatment algorithm

7.7 Long-term treatment

GAD patients often require long-term treatment as many patients experience persistent symptoms over time. As previously noted, response with first-line agents can continue to accrue over 6 to 12 months or longer of treatment. Unfortunately, in spite of adequate treatment, ~20% to 40% or more of GAD patients will relapse within 6 months of medication discontinuation. As well, several controlled relapse prevention studies have shown significantly lower rates of relapse by staying on medication versus being switched to placebo. Long-term medication use may be required to prevent relapse. CBT may be a more enduring treatment as open-label follow-up studies have demonstrated that the benefits of CBT treatment can be sustained for 1 to 2 yrs post-treatment, although this remains to be confirmed in randomized controlled trial (Bandelow *et al.*, 2008).

7.8 Treating GAD in special populations

7.8.1 Pregnancy and breastfeeding

As GAD often affects women during their child-bearing age, considerations regarding pregnancy and breastfeeding need to be taken into account as part of treatment planning. Unfortunately no decision regarding treatment during pregnancy or breastfeeding is without risk and the reader is referred to more specialized resources (e.g. Massachusetts General Hospital Center for Womens Mental Health, Boston, http://www.womensmentalhealth.org/; The Hospital for Sick Children, Toronto, www.motherisk.org) for a comprehensive review of these issues and should seek consultation with local specialists (e.g. ob-gyn) when appropriate for discussion regarding a particular patient. The decision to treat or not includes consideration of the mother's level of distress, ability to adequately care for herself during the pre- and postnatal period, and unknown effects of maternal anxiety and stress on the developing foetus and baby. In general, psychosocial therapies, if effective may be preferable to pharmacotherapy by minimizing foetal exposure; however, many individuals may not have access to CBT, while others may present already on medication and may require more urgent intervention.

Although this remains an area requiring more study, the use of antidepressants in pregnancy, particularly the SSRIs and TCAs, does not appear to cause an increased risk of major birth defects, with the exception of paroxetine which may have a twofold increase in the risk of major birth defects, including cardiac septal defects as compared to other SSRIs. However, the use of SSRIs (the whole class of agents) during pregnancy has been associated with a sixfold increase in risk of pulmonary abnormalities (persistent pulmonary hypertension) in infants. First trimester benzodiazepine exposure may be associated with an increased risk of cleft lip (<1 in 1,000 cases).

The use of antidepressants during pregnancy can lead to drug discontinuation syndrome (e.g. tremors and irritability) in the newborn through parturition. Although data addressing this issue are limited, prenatal exposure to antidepressants does not seem to affect cognition, language development, or temperament in children, with the best studied agents being fluoxetine and the TCAs. Prenatal use of high-dose benzodiazepines has been associated with a withdrawal syndrome in the newborn characterized by symptoms of irritability, restlessness, apnoea, cyanosis, lethargy, and hypotonia (Menon, 2008; Nordeng and Spigset, 2005).

An important principle for the maternal use of medications during breastfeeding is to avoid using excessively sedating antidepressants. The risks of the adverse events in the infant need to be assessed on a case-by-case basis; however, consultation with expert resources is imperative (e.g. Massachusetts General Hospital Center for Womens Mental Health, Boston, http://www.womensmentalhealth.org/; The Hospital for Sick Children, Toronto, www.motherisk.org). Most antidepressants including the SSRIs and the TCAs are excreted into the breast milk. Plasma levels of the SSRIs, sertraline and paroxetine, as well as the TCA, nortriptyline, are virtually undetectable in breastfed infants and may be the preferred agents when breastfeeding.

The issue of medication use in pregnancy and breastfeeding is an evolving area, so it is critical to consult current resources in helping patients make informed choices regarding their therapeutic options.

7.9 Treatment in children and adolescents

GAD may have its onset in childhood. Although the GAD criteria for children are the same as in adults, children may present differently with somatic complaints such as stomach aches and headaches, crying, and nightmares. Children are often unaware of their worries and can be hard pressed to verbalize them. They often do not see their worries as excessive and uncontrollable. GAD may present co-morbidly in childhood with separation anxiety disorder and social phobia. Assessment of the child/adolescent ideally requires multiple informants including the parents, teacher, and child as the anxiety may present differently in different environments. Standardized questionnaires such as the Multidimensional Anxiety Scale for Children (MASC) and the Screen for Child Anxiety Related Disorders (SCARED) may assist in the diagnosis and are helpful in monitoring treatment response. Treatment of childhood GAD usually starts with education and support. Psychological treatment in the form of CBT is typically initiated first. CBT for children needs to be adapted to the child's age and developmental status and is generally presented in a simpler and more concrete manner. Parental involvement seems to enhance outcomes. In general, pharmacotherapy is not used alone but is often added to CBT or other psychosocial interventions, even though the combination has not been well studied. The risks and benefits of medications need to be assessed on a case-by-case basis. Antidepressants in the form of SSRIs are the first-line medication treatment in children. Dosing is highly variable and therefore requires initiation at very low doses with a very slow upward titration that can end up in the adult dosing range. Potential side effects include gastrointestinal, anxiety, agitation, and overactivation. In addition, the possibility that antidepressant exposure may precipitate a cardinal manic or hypo manic episode in a previously undiagnosed bipolar child or adolescent should be recognized. The potential risk of SSRI-induced suicidality has been primarily studied in depression. Although the risk for suicidality in non-depression studies was higher than placebo, the attributable risk for serious suicidal events was less than in depression studies and in fact was not statistically significant from placebo. Although it remains an area requiring further study, the association of antidepressants and suicidality in children and adolescents should be borne in mind and monitored.

7.10 Treatment in the elderly

Anxiety symptoms are common in the elderly; however, most anxiety disorders including GAD have their onset earlier in adulthood, and persist into old age. Although late onset GAD has been reported in elderly populations, there is an age decline in prevalence as with other anxiety disorders between the ages of 65 and 85, and newly emergent anxiety symptoms in late life should raise consideration of potential medical/medication causes as well as the presence of other psychiatric conditions including depression and dementia. GAD in late life is usually co-morbid with other psychiatric conditions, particularly major depression. The presentation of late onset GAD is often characterized by the absence of uncontrollable worry. Rather, the elderly present with somatic complaints, feelings of tension, and anxious mood, which can be layered on top of a concurrent major depression or dementia. To make a diagnosis of GAD in the elderly, the clinician needs to obtain a thorough psychiatric history and mental status examination of the patient, as well as history from the patient's family and caregivers. In addition, the elderly patient may require a physical examination and laboratory tests to rule out potential underlying medical conditions as well as an evaluation of alcohol and substance use. Due to the high prevalence of medical conditions and use of prescription medications in the elderly, the diagnosis of

GAD is often not straightforward. As well, the elderly face a number of stressful life changes associated with aging, including financial changes with retirement, diminished cognitive functioning and physical health, and changes in personal relationships through the death of spouse or friends. All of these important issues can add challenges to making the diagnosis of GAD in the elderly. Elderly GAD patients tend to focus more on finances, social and interpersonal issues, and personal health as compared to elderly individuals without GAD. Differentiating realistic worries of late life from GAD requires an evaluation of the frequency, intensity, duration, and controllability of the worry as well as the impairment and distress caused by the worry.

Interventions should include a psychoeducational programme for the patient and family as well as possible enhancements to the patient's social, recreational, and spiritual environment. Psychological treatments for late-life GAD have had only a limited evaluation. CBT has been found to be efficacious in this population although response rates are typically lower than that has been found in younger GAD populations. Supportive therapy has been found to be equally effective to CBT in some studies of elderly GAD. CBT for elderly GAD will likely require adaptation, by using age appropriate learning strategies such as the use of memory aids, cross-modal repetition, and frequent summarizing.

There have been only a limited number of randomized controlled trials of pharmacotherapy in the elderly. The elderly often show an increased sensitivity to side effects of psychotropic agents due to age-related changes in physiology. Antimuscarinic side effects, somnolence, orthostatic hypotension, electrocardiogram (ECG) changes, extra-pyramidal effects, amnestic and other cognitive and paradoxical effects with benzodiazepines, as well as benzodiazepine withdrawal and dependence are common sensitivities seen in this population. As the elderly are often taking several medications, there is the potential for drug interactions which needs to be taken into consideration when choosing a medication. Given the frequent co-morbidity with depression and concerns about potential adverse effects on memory and cognition with benzodiazepines in the elderly, antidepressants, typically the SSRIs, are generally considered appropriate first-line interventions for elderly anxious patients. Augmentation or alternative treatment with buspirone, anticonvulsants, and atypicals or benzodiazepines may be considered if needed with careful attention to issues of dosing giving the increased sensitivity of the elderly to side effects. Medication needs to be initiated at the lowest possible dose and increases should be slow and gradual; thus it may take elderly patients longer to see significant therapeutic benefit, and they should be informed of this at initiation of treatment.

References

Baldwin DS, Anderson IM, Nutt DJ *et al.* (2005). Evidence-based guidelines for the pharmacological treatment of anxiety disorders: recommendations from the British Association for Psychopharmacology. *J Psychopharm*, **19**, 567–96.

Bandelow B, Zohar J, Hollander E, Kasper S, Moller HJ, WFSBP Task Force. (2008). World Federation of Societies of Biological Psychiatry (WFSBP) Guidelines for the Pharmacological Treatment of Anxiety, Obsessive Compulsive and Post-traumatic Stress Disorders—First Revision. *World J Biol Psychiatry*, **9** (4), 248–312.

Canadian Psychiatric Association. (2006). Clinical practice guidelines: management of anxiety disorders. *Can J Psych*, **51** (Suppl 2), 1S–92S.

Menon SJ. (2008). Psychotropic medication during pregnancy and lactation. *Arch Gynecol Obstet*, **277**, 1–13.

Nordeng H, Spigset O. (2005). Treatment with selective serotonin reuptake inhibitors in the third trimester of pregnancy. Effects on the infant. *Drug Safety*, **28** (7), 565–81.

Chapter 8

Self-help resources

Michael Van Ameringen and Mark H. Pollack

> **Key point**
> • Self-help resources can be effective tools to enhance treatment of generalized anxiety disorder (GAD).

8.1 Introduction

Self-help treatments are frequently used in the treatment of anxiety disorders. Media such as self-help books, treatment manuals, audio tapes, Internet sites, and computer programs can be very useful tools for patients and require little assistance from a therapist or clinician. Using these types of treatments while engaged in psychotherapy has been shown to decrease the number of visits to the therapist. Several studies have also indicated that the efficacy of self-help treatments for anxiety disorders rivals that of therapist-led treatments.

Patients with generalized anxiety disorder (GAD) often seek help for the physical symptoms associated with their disorder or for co-morbid psychiatric conditions such as depression or panic disorder rather than for GAD itself. The tendency for individuals with GAD to try to 'cope with the symptoms on their own' has been well-documented in the literature. GAD patients often turn to self-help treatments and most often chose audio tapes and books. In the small number of studies which have examined the efficacy of self-help treatments in GAD, the findings have been positive with one study showing treatment gains maintained for up to 2 yrs.

We have compiled a list of helpful books and Internet sites specifically related to GAD.

8.2 Books

Women Who Worry Too Much. Holly Hazlett-Stevens (2005). Oakland, CA: New Harbinger Publications, ISBN: 1572244127.

Ten Simple Solutions to Worry. Kevin Gyoerkoe and Pamela Wiegartz (2006). Oakland, CA: New Harbinger Publications, ISBN: 1572244658.

Solving Life's Problems: A 5-Step Guide to Enhanced Well-Being. Arthur M. Nezu, Christine Maguth Nezu, and Thomas D'Zurilla (2006). New York, NY: Springer Publishing Company, ISBN-10: 082611489X.

10 Simple Solutions to Stress: How to Tame Tension and Start Enjoying Your Life. Claire Michaels Wheeler (2007). Oakland, CA: New Harbinger Publications, ISBN-13: 978-157224476-4.

The Anxiety and Phobia Workbook, Third Edition. Bourne EJ (1995). Oakland, CA: New Harbinger Publications, ISBN 157224223X.

Worry Control Workbook. Copland E (1998). Oakland, CA: New Harbinger Publications, ISBN 1572241209.

8.3 **Audio books**

The Worry Cure: Seven Steps to Stop Worry from Stopping You (2006) Robert L. Leahy and Mike Chamberlain—Abridged.

The Worrywart's Companion: Twenty-One Ways to Soothe Yourself and Worry Smart (1998) Beverly Potter and Kitt Weagant—Abridged.

How to Stop Worrying and Start Living (1999) Dale Carnegie.

8.4 **Websites**

www.anxietybc.com: Self-help information and programs, as well as resources for parents and caregivers.

www.adaa.org: Anxiety Disorders Association of America.

www.nimh.nih.gov/health/topics/generalized-anxiety-disorder-gad/index.shtml: The National Institute of Mental Health.

www.anxieties.com: Brief self-help resources for a variety of anxiety disorders.

www.anxietycanada.ca: Anxiety Disorders Association of Canada.

www.massgeneral.org/allpsych/anxiety/index.asp: The Center for Anxiety and Traumatic Stress Disorders, Massachusetts General Hospital.

www.macanxiety.com: Anxiety Disorders Clinic, McMaster University Medical Centre, Canada.

www.nopanic.org.uk: A UK charitable organization which offers telephone support and self-help materials for anxiety disorders.

www.anxietyuk.org.uk: Anxiety UK, a self-help organization.

Appendix

Rating Scales for GAD

GAD-7

1. Feeling nervous, anxious, or on edge?
   0 = not at all
   1 = several days
   2 = more than half the days
   3 = nearly everyday
2. Not being able to stop or control worrying?
   0 = not at all
   1 = several days
   2 = more than half the days
   3 = nearly everyday
3. Worrying too much about different things?
   0 = not at all
   1 = several days
   2 = more than half the days
   3 = nearly everyday
4. Trouble relaxing?
   0 = not at all
   1 = several days
   2 = more than half the days
   3 = nearly everyday
5. Being so restless that it is hard to sit still?
   0 = not at all
   1 = several days
   2 = more than half the days
   3 = nearly everyday
6. Becoming easily annoyed or irritable?
   0 = not at all
   1 = several days
   2 = more than half the days
   3 = nearly everyday
7. Feeling afraid as if something awful might happen?
   0 = not at all
   1 = several days
   2 = more than half the days
   3 = nearly everyday

If you checked off any problems, how difficult have these problems made it for you to do your work, take care of things at home, or get along with other people?

__ Not difficult at all   __ Somewhat difficult

__ Very difficult   __ Extremely difficult

Scoring: Add the results for question number one through seven to get a total score. If you score 10 or above you might want to consider one or more of the following: discuss your symptoms with your doctor, contact a local mental health-care provider, or contact my office for further assessment and possible treatment. Although these questions serve as a useful guide, only an appropriate licensed health professional can make the diagnosis of GAD.

Adapted from: Spitzer RL, Kroenke K, Williams JBW, Lowe B. (2006). A brief measure for assessing generalized anxiety disorder. *Arch Inter Med*, **166**, 1092–7.

Penn State Worry Questionnaire

Instructions: Please rate the following statements using the scale below.

1	2	3	4	5
Not at all typical of me				Very typical of me

1. If I do not have enough time to do everything, I do not worry about it _____
2. My worries overwhelm me _____
3. I do not tend to worry about things _____
4. Many situations make me worry _____
5. I know I should not worry about things, but I just cannot help it _____
6. When I am under pressure I worry a lot _____
7. I am always worrying about something _____
8. I find it easy to dismiss worrisome thoughts _____
9. As soon as I finish one task, I start to worry about everything else have to do _____
10. I never worry about anything _____
11. When there is nothing more I can do about a concern, I do not worry about it any more _____
12. I have been a worrier all my life _____
13. I notice that I have been worrying about things _____
14. Once I start worrying, I cannot stop _____
15. I worry all the time _____
16. I worry about projects until they are all done _____

Adapted from: Meyer TJ, Miller ML, Metzger RL, Borkovec TD. (1990). Development and validation of the Penn State Worry Questionnaire. *Behav Res Ther*, **28**, 487–95.

Depression Anxiety Stress Scales (DASS₍₂₁₎)

Please read each statement and circle a number 0, 1, 2, or 3 that indicates how much the statement applied to you *over the past week*. There are no right or wrong answers. Do not spend too much time on any statement.

The rating scale is as follows:

0   Did not apply to me at all
1   Applied to me to some degree, or some of the time
2   Applied to me to a considerable degree, or a good part of time
3   Applied to me very much, or most of the time

1	I found it hard to wind down	0	1	2	3
2	I was aware of dryness of my mouth	0	1	2	3
3	I couldn't seem to experience any positive feeling at all	0	1	2	3
4	I experienced breathing difficulty (eg, excessively rapid breathing, breathlessness in the absence of physical exertion)	0	1	2	3
5	I found it difficult to work up the initiative to do things	0	1	2	3
6	I tended to over-react to situations	0	1	2	3
7	I experienced trembling (eg, in the hands)	0	1	2	3
8	I felt that I was using a lot of nervous energy	0	1	2	3
9	I was worried about situations in which I might panic and make a fool of myself	0	1	2	3
10	I felt that I had nothing to look forward to	0	1	2	3
11	I found myself getting agitated	0	1	2	3
12	I found it difficult to relax	0	1	2	3
13	I felt down-hearted and blue	0	1	2	3
14	I was intolerant of anything that kept me from getting on with what I was doing	0	1	2	3
15	I felt I was close to panic	0	1	2	3
16	I was unable to become enthusiastic about anything	0	1	2	3
17	I felt I wasn't worth much as a person	0	1	2	3
18	I felt that I was rather touchy	0	1	2	3
19	I was aware of the action of my heart in the absence of physical exertion (eg, sense of heart rate increase, heart missing a beat)	0	1	2	3
20	I felt scared without any good reason	0	1	2	3
21	I felt that life was meaningless	0	1	2	3

Lovibond SH, Lovibond PF. *Manual for the Depression Anxiety Stress Scales*, 1995. Sydney NSW. The Psychology Foundation of Australia.

Intolerance of Uncertainly Scale (IUS)

You will find below a series of statements which describe how people may react to the uncertainties of life. Please use the scale below to describe to what extent each item is a characteristic of you. Please enter a number (1 to 5) that describes you best.

1	2	3	4	5
Not at all Characteristic of me		Somewhat Characteristic of me		Entirely Characteristic of me

1. _____ Uncertainty stops me from having a firm opinion
2. _____ Being uncertain means that a person is disorganized
3. _____ Uncertainty makes life intolerable
4. _____ It's unfair not having any guarantees in life
5. _____ My mind can't be relaxed if I don't know what will happen tomorrow
6. _____ Uncertainty makes me uneasy, anxious, or stressed
7. _____ Unforeseen events upset me greatly
8. _____ It frustrates me not having all the information I need
9. _____ Uncertainty keeps me from living a full life
10. _____ One should always look ahead so as to avoid surprises
11. _____ A small unforeseen event can spoil everything, even with the best of planning
12. _____ When it's time to act, uncertainty paralyses me
13. _____ Being uncertain means that I am not first rate
14. _____ When I am uncertain, I can't go forward
15. _____ When I am uncertain, I can't function very well
16. _____ Unlike me, others always seem to know where they are going with their lives
17. _____ Uncertainty makes me vulnerable, unhappy, or sad
18. _____ I always want to know what the future has in store for me
19. _____ I can't stand being taken by surprise
20. _____ The smallest doubt can stop me from acting
21. _____ I should be able to organize everything in advance
22. _____ Being uncertain means that I lack confidence
23. _____ I think it's unfair that other people seem sure about their future
24. _____ Uncertainty keeps me from sleeping soundly
25. _____ I must get away from all uncertain situations
26. _____ The ambiguities in life stress me
27. _____ I can't stand being undecided about my future[*]

* Reprinted from Buhr K, Dugas MJ. (2002). The intolerance of Uncertainty Scale: psychometric properties of the English version. *Behav Res Ther*, **40**, 931–45 (with permission from Elsevier).

Hamilton anxiety scale (HAM-A)**

Item	Cue	Not present (0)	Mild (1)	Moderate (2)	Severe (3)	Very severe (4)
1. Anxious mood	Worries, anticipation of the worst, fearful anticipation, irritability					
2. Tension	Feelings of tension, fatigability, startle response, moves to tears easily, trembling, feeling of restlessness, inability to relax					
3. Fears	Of dark, of strangers, of being left alone, of animals, of traffic, of crowds, etc.					
4. Insomnia	Difficulty in falling asleep, broken sleep, unsatisfying sleep and fatigue on waking, dreams, nightmares, night terrors					
5. Intellectual (cognitive)	Difficulty in concentration, poor memory					
6. Depressed mood	Loss of interest, lack of pleasure in hobbies, depression, early waking, diurnal swings					
7. Somatic (muscular)	Pains and aches, twitching, stiffness, myoclonic jerks, grinding of teeth, unsteady voice, increased muscular tone					

8. Somatic (sensory)	Tinnitus, blurring of vision, hot and cold flushes, feelings of weakness, pricking sensation
9. Cardiovascular symptoms	Tachycardia, palpitations, pain in chest, throbbing in vessels, fainting feelings, missing beat
10. Respiratory symptoms	Pressure or constriction in chest, choking feelings, sighing, dyspnoea
11. Gastrointestinal symptoms	Difficulty in swallowing, wind, abdominal pain, burning sensations, abdominal fullness, nausea, vomiting, borborygmi, looseness of bowels, loss of weight, constipation
12. Genitourinary symptoms	Frequency of micturition, urgency of micturition, amenorrhea, menorrhagia, development of frigidity, premature ejaculation, loss of libido, impotence
13. Autonomic symptoms	Dry mouth, flushing, pallor, tendency to sweat, giddiness, tension, headache, raising of hair
14. Behaviour at interview	Fidgeting, restlessness or pacing, tremor of hands, furrowed brow, strained face, sighing or rapid respiration, facial pallor, swallowing, belching, brisk tendon jerks, dilated pupils, exophthalmos

** Adapted from: Hamilton M. (1959). The assessment of anxiety states by rating. *Br J Med Psych*, **32**, 50–5

Generalized Anxiety Disorder Severity Scale (GADSS)

Target worry list	Rated as yes or no; if yes, specific worry is listed in comment field	Not scored
Future; own health; other's health; family well-being; finances; social relationships; intimate relationships; work; school; routine daily activities; other		
Target worry	Rater lists one or two target worries	Target worries used in first question of the scored section
Item	**Script**	**Scoring anchors**
Frequency of worries	How often do you worry about (list target worry)? Do you worry all day long? Do you worry every day? On average, how much of each day did you have one or more of these symptoms?	0 No worries 1 Slight—worry occupies <1 h per day 2 Moderate—worries for 1 to 3 h per day 3 Severe—worries occur 3 to 8 h per day 4 Very severe—>8 h of worry per day
Distress due to worrying	How much distress does worrying cause you? How upset or uncomfortable do you feel when you are worrying?	0 None 1 Mild, not too disturbing 2 Moderate, definitely disturbing but still manageable 3 Severe, very intense, and disturbing 4 Very severe, incapacitating

Frequency of associated symptoms (restlessness, feeling keyed up or on edge, irritability, muscle tension, difficulty concentrating, mind going blank, fatigue, sleep disturbance)	Over the past week, how often did you experience these symptoms? Did you have these symptoms every day? On average, during how much of each day did you have one or more of these symptoms?	0 Not at all 1 Slightly—symptoms present <1 h per day 2 Moderate—symptoms for 1 to 3 h per day 3 Severe—symptoms occur 3 to 8 h per day 4 Very severe—symptoms are present >8 h per day
Severity and distress due to associated symptoms	During the past week, on average, when you had these symptoms, how intense were they? How much distress did these symptoms cause you? How upset or uncomfortable did you feel when you had them?	0 None 1 Mild, noticeably but not too intense or disturbing 2 Moderate, definitely disturbing but still manageable 3 Severe, very, very intense, and disturbing 4 Very severe, incapacitating
Impairment/interference in work functioning	How much do the symptoms we have been discussing interfere with your ability to work and/or carry out responsibilities at home—or ability to get things done as quickly and effectively? Are there things you are not doing because of your anxiety? Does anxiety ever cause you to take short cuts or request assistance to get thing done?	0 None 1 Mild, slight interference, but overall performance not affected 2 Moderate, definite interference but still manageable 3 Severe, causes substantial impairment 4 Very severe, incapacitating

Item	Script	Scoring anchors
Impairment/interference in social functioning	How much do the symptoms we have been discussing interfere with your social life? Are you spending less time with friends and relatives than you used to? Do you turn down requests of opportunities to socialize? Are there certain restrictions in your social life about where or how long you will socialize?	0 None 1 Mild, slight interference, but overall performance not affected 2 Moderate, definite interference but still manageable 3 Severe, causes substantial impairment 4 Very severe, incapacitating

Adapted from: Shear K, Belnap BH, Mazumdar S, Houck P, Rollman BL. (2006). Generalized anxiety disorder severity scale: a preliminary validation study. *Depress Anx*, **23**, 77–82.

Index

NB: Page numbers in *italics* relate to Boxes, Figures or Tables